UNDERSTANDING YOUR HORSE

SKIN DISEASES
of the Horse

Understanding
your Horse

UNDERSTANDING YOUR HORSE

ANKE RÜSBÜLDT

SKIN DISEASES
of the Horse

Prevention • Diagnosis • Treatment

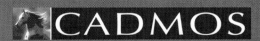

Copyright © 2007 by Cadmos Verlag GmbH, Schwarzenbek, Germany
Copyright of this edition © 2010 by Cadmos Books, Great Britain
English translation: Ute Weyer
Title Photograph: Sabine Stuewer
Layout: Ravenstein + Partner, Verden, Germany
Photographs: Ilka Hoppe, Sabine Struewer, Christiane Slawik
Editorial: Anneke Bosse, Dr Sarah Binns, Christopher Long
Printed by: Westermann Druck, Zwickau
British Library Cataloguing in Publication Data
A catalogue record of this book is available from the British Library.

Printed in Germany

ISBN 978-3-86127-978-5

www.cadmos.co.uk

Contents

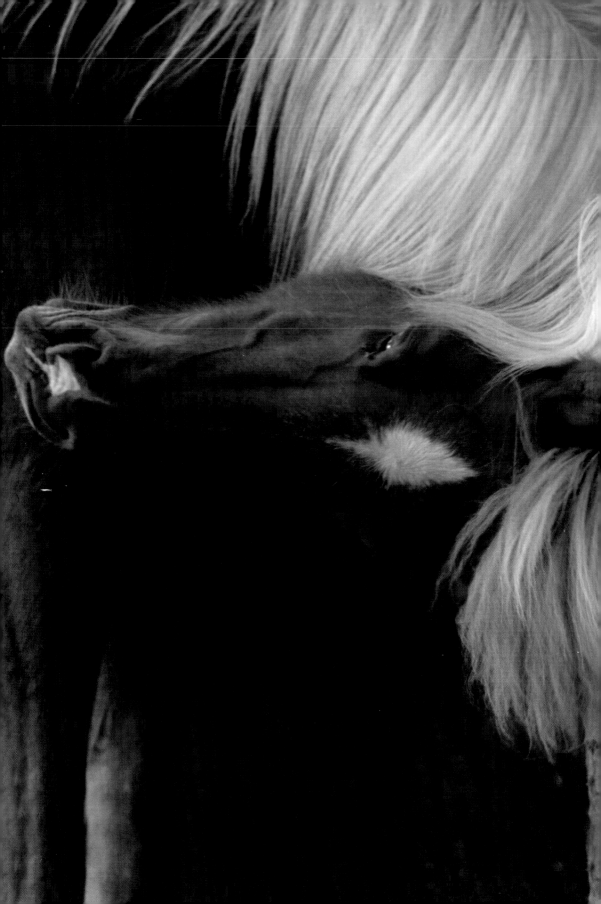

Contents

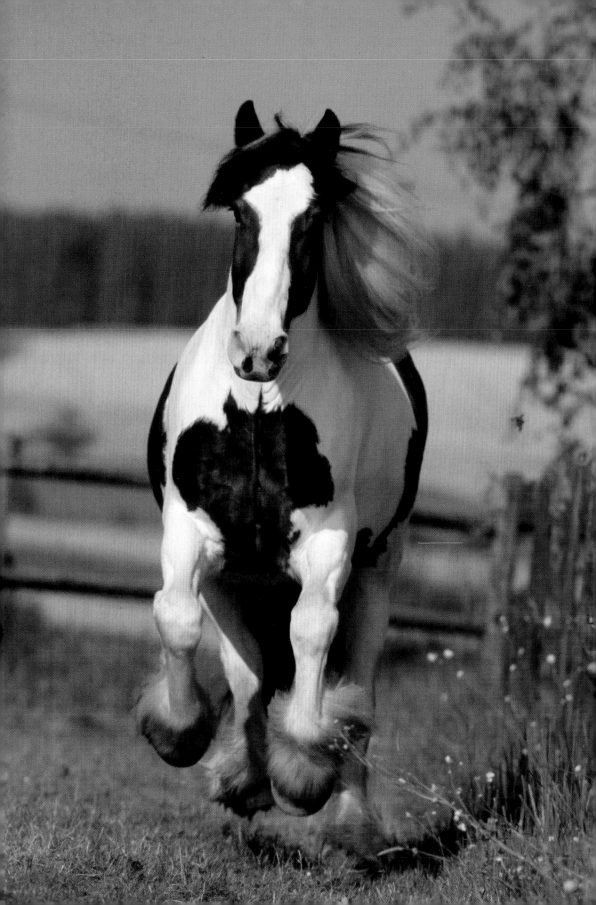

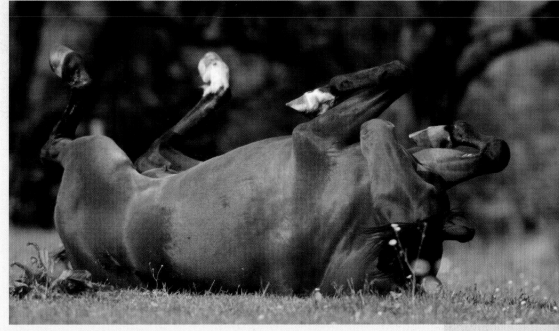

A shiny coat is a sign of healthy skin as well as mental well-being. (Photo Stuewer)

Introduction

Skin diseases in horses are unpopular among veterinary surgeons, horse owners and the horses themselves. There are far more questions than answers. Correct diagnosis of a skin disease is often diffi-cult to determine, and treatments are frequently lengthy and often unsatis-factory. This book offers an overview of the most common skin diseases and provides guidance for their sensible management. It is crucial to recognise the type of skin disease, to understand which further diagnostic measures should be carried out, and finally to know the best treatment regime to apply.

Mucous membranes – for example those inside the mouth and around the eyes – have a similar structure to the outer skin and react in similar ways. This book, however, is limited to problems of the outer skin and does not deal with diseases of the mucous membranes. Hoof problems are also too broad a subject for this book; this topic is covered in dedica-ted books such as *No Foot, No Horse: Foot Balance* by Gail Williams and Martin Deacon, *Kenilworth Press*.

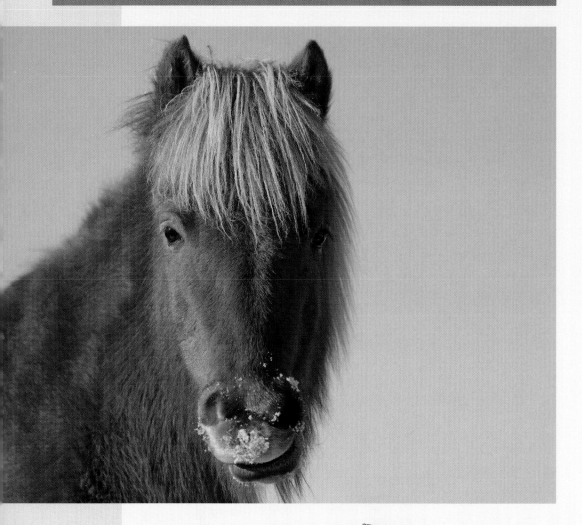

The skin

The skin is the largest organ of the body. It is the outer shell and provides a barrier against external influences. The skin regulates temperature, produces sweat and provides the coat or fur. It is also an important tactile organ, sensing temperature, pressure and pain.

The skin protects the body from the ingress of living organisms (e.g. bacteria), as well as from physical influences such as heat or radiation. The skin contains immune cells which are part of the specific and non-specific immune defences. Glands in the skin produce various substances; one example is grease, which has protective qualities. The skin pigments offer protection from sunlight and the skin is involved in body fluid regulation. Subcutaneous fat shapes the body and also acts as a shock absorber and energy store. The skin manufactures essential substances, such as vitamin D, by using sunlight. Therefore the skin plays an important role in the metabolism of the whole body.

Furthermore, not only the facial expression but also the appearance of the skin mirrors the animal's health.

Structure of the skin

The skin consists of two main layers – the epidermis and dermis – beneath which lies the subcutaneous tissue. The epidermis is formed mainly from epidermal cells, but also contains melanocytes (which protect against light, and colour the skin), immune cells and tactile cells.

Microscopically we can distinguish four layers. On the outside lie the keratinocytes (forming the stratum corneum) which produce a horn-like protein called keratin. Beneath the keratinocytes is a

The skin is a complex organ with many functions. (Drawing: Retsch-Amschler)

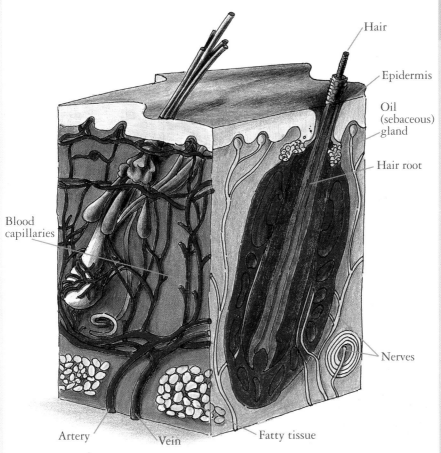

Hair

Epidermis

Oil (sebaceous) gland

Hair root

Nerves

Blood capillaries

Artery

Vein

Fatty tissue

layer of cells containing a very fine grid (the stratum granulosum), and beneath the stratum granulosum lies the spinous or 'prickle-cell' layer (stratum spinosum). The lowest layer is called the stratum basale.

The dermis is formed predominantly of connective tissue. It contains hair follicles and glands. Hair and the exit ducts of the glands cross through this layer.

Each hair is produced inside a hair follicle. Apart from the mane and tail hairs and the tactile hairs around the muzzle and eyes, all hairs that make up the coat are of the same length and stability, unlike those of animals that have an undercoat. During moulting the new hair grows from the follicle and pushes the old hair out.

A small gland is attached along the side of each hair follicle which produces an oily type of sweat that coats the hair. This oily substance has antibacterial properties and also covers the skin with a protective layer. Sweat glands are distributed all over the skin (up to 100 glands per square centimetre of skin surface).

Sweat production is an essential part of the thermoregulatory system of the body, but the glands also help to eliminate waste products and send out pheromones.

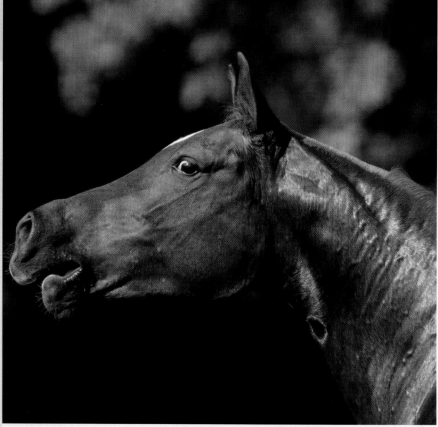

Sweating enables the horse to regulate its body temperature. (Photo: Stuewer)

The dermis is well supplied with blood vessels, which are organised in loops and connected with each other throughout the different skin layers. These blood vessels are an essential part of the body's thermoregulatory system. Infections or traumatic processes increase the circulation of blood.

Also located in the skin are melanocytes (which define the skin colour) and numerous immune cells. Furthermore, free nerve endings reach into the layers of the dermis. Some stem from the central nervous system and innervate the hair follicles, thus triggering raising of the hair as a response to certain stimuli. Other nerves send information from the skin to the central nervous system, for example the sensation of cold. These nerve impulses are autonomic, meaning they cannot be influenced consciously. It is the same for us – we cannot raise the hairs on our arms willingly, but when we are cold they are raised automatically.

A horse can detect very fine stimuli with its skin, such as a fly landing on its back. An impulse is then sent to the skin muscles: the skin twitches and the fly takes off. These reflexes happen very quickly because the nerve impulses are sent via the spinal cord within a split second.

The free nerve endings are all fine branches that stem from the main spinal cord nerves. The only exception is the innervation of the facial skin via the fifth cranial nerve, the trigeminal nerve.

The subcutis (subcutaneous layer) is an effective fat storage area. It also contains muscle fibres that allow isolated skin contractions, as we can see when an insects lands on the skin.

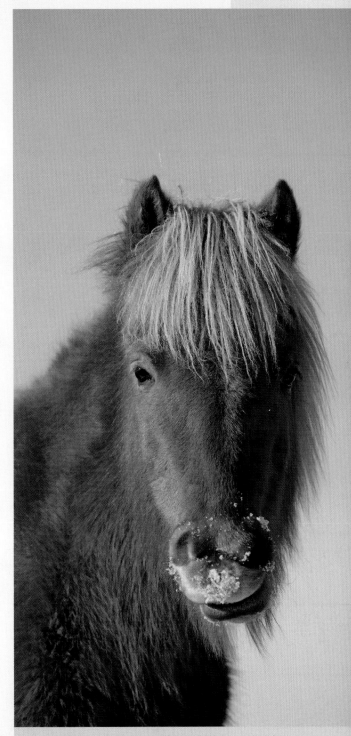

Nerve endings that innervate the hair follicles send information about skin temperature to the brain thus causing the hairs to stand up.
(Photo: Slawik)

The coat

When looking at a horse its coat really stands out, especially a shiny summer coat.

Healthy horses have a natural sheen whether they have been groomed or not, because healthy hair is smooth and lies flat over the skin. An even distribution of oil and sweat from the skin glands encourages the shiny appearance.

An unhealthy horse raises its hair slightly because it feels unwell or cold and the coat then appears rough and uneven. A lack of certain vitamins or insufficient nutrition can cause hair to break or fall out and the natural sheen is then lost. Lack of vitamins can also lead to the development of dandruff, or scurf.

When they are moulting, horses can often look scruffy.

Moulting during spring and autumn is a great challenge for the body's metabolism because the hair of the past season falls out and the whole coat is replaced.

Some horses change their colour during the moult (e.g. some black horses appear brown in the winter).

During moulting the horse requires more proteins and vitamins and any nutritional deficiencies can create even greater problems than at other times.

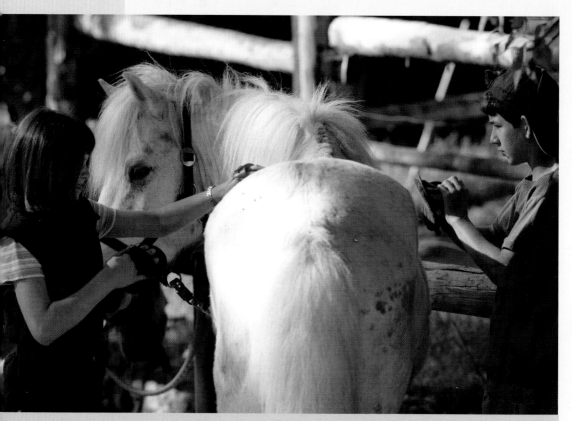

Grooming is important but only within reason: too much can damage the skin and coat. (Photo: Slawik)

Overview of skin diseases

Skin diseases can have infectious or non-infectious causes. Often both types occur together, because traumatised skin is more susceptible to secondary infections, or one infection may allow other agents to damage the skin further.

Different skin diseases can develop at the same time. Owing to the limited response mechanisms of the skin many diseases have a very similar range of clinical signs.

Infectious skin diseases

Infectious skin diseases are diseases caused by a living organism that enters the body, replicates itself and causes specific clinical signs. The different organisms can be distinguished by their pathogenicity, that is, their ability to cause disease. Whether they cause disease at all also depends on the body's susceptibility to them. These agents are often one of a multitude of factors causing a disease. For example, bacteria can cause infections more easily in skin that has been damaged previously by burns.

The different types of organism are:
• **Viruses:** viruses are minute organisms without their own metabolism. They depend on the metabolism of their hosts — body cells or bacteria. Common viral skin diseases include sarcoids (for which a viral cause is most likely), warts (papilloma virus) and pox.
• **Bacteria:** bacteria are pathogens that consist of a single cell. Some of the bacterial diseases that we deal with are dermatophilosis, folliculitis (infection of hair follicles) and furunculosis.

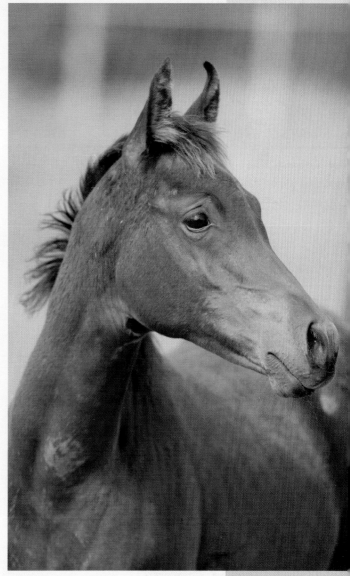

Many skin diseases have similar appearances — diagnosis is not always easy. (Photo: Slawik)

• **Fungi:** fungal diseases are among the most common skin complaints in horses. These organisms are multicellular and produce spores.
• **Parasites:** more complex organisms can also cause skin diseases, for example mites, ticks and lice. Certain worms can affect the skin, although they play a greater role in intestinal problems.

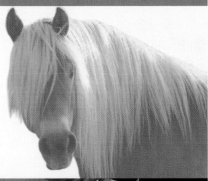

Non-infectious skin diseases

This category includes all other causes: nutritional, environmental, traumatic, hereditary, immunological (e.g. allergies) and hormonal diseases (e.g. Cushing's syndrome), and tumours.

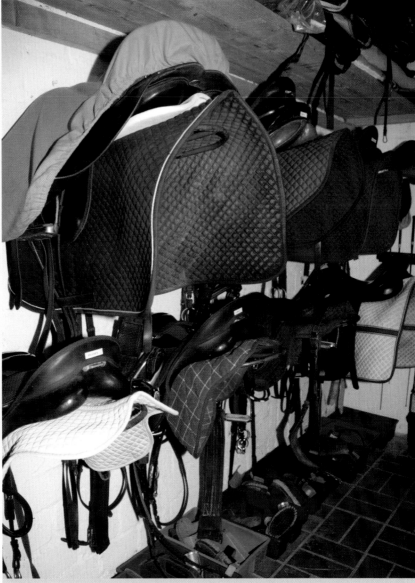

In order to prevent the spread of skin disease from one horse to another, each horse should have its own tack and grooming kit. (Photo: Slawik)

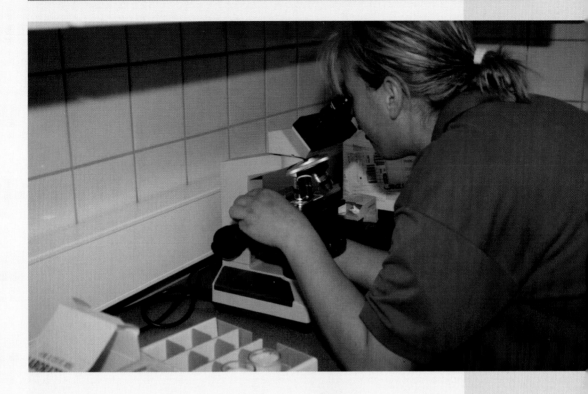

Diagnosis of skin diseases

Diagnosis and treatment of skin diseases in horses should be carried out by a veterinary surgeon. Be very careful when trying to diagnose or treat skin diseases yourself!

Sometimes the wrong initial treatment can make the situation a lot worse and the consulting vet will often not be able to correct these mistaken diagnoses at a later stage. Treated skin can also alter any diagnostic results. For the welfare of your horse, it is better to consult the vet first.

Disease history

An important step towards a successful diagnosis is observation and a detailed disease history.

The history should include age, breed, sex and colour of the horse as this information can often give important clues to the problem.

Some diseases only occur in unpigmented skin, or affect a certain age group more than others.

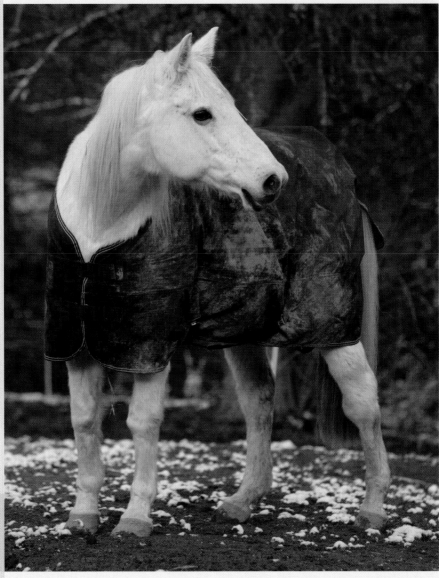

Does the horse wear a rug in winter? Questions such as this are an important part of the animal's history. (Photo: Slawik)

The history also establishes how long the problem has been present, what it looked like in the early stages and whether other body parts or other horses are affected. It is very important to know whether the lesions are itching.

Other information such as details of husbandry can also give clues. Does the horse wear a rug, does it rub, does it share its tack with other horses?

The vaccination history and worm management should also be mentioned. For a mare, the phase of the oestrous cycle and potential pregnancy are important.

Some tail rubbing during her season or oedema in late pregnancy is normal and not a skin disease.

What is pruritus?

Pruritus (itchiness) is the key sign of many skin diseases. It can be caused by external influences transmitted through the sensitive innervation of the skin, or it can originate from within the skin through the release of trigger substances from the cells (inflammatory mediators).

One of these substances is histamine. Histamine is usually retained in certain immune cells, for example mast cells. When a pathological agent meets antibodies located on the surfaces of the mast cells the cells release histamine, which then triggers a cascade of reactions in the skin – one of which is pruritus.

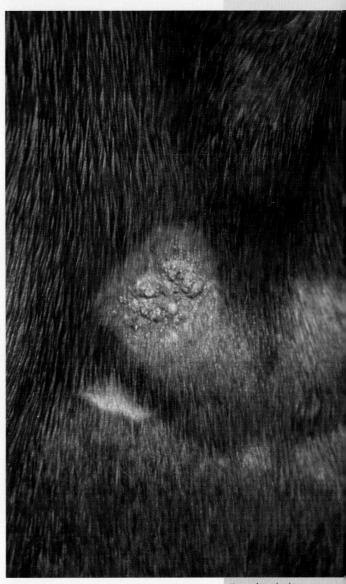

As much as the skin lesions claim our attention, examination of the whole horse is important. (Photo: Stuewer)

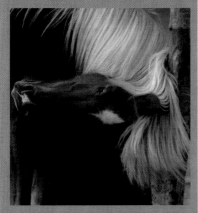

Many skin diseases cause itchiness through the release of histamine. (Photo: Stuewer)

Clinical examination

Once the vet has established a detailed disease history the horse needs to be examined. It is important to examine the whole horse briefly in order not to miss any underlying problems. Some skin diseases do not affect the well-being of the horse very much but are a nuisance in the opinion of the owner. Extensive therapy with significant side effects may not be an option in these cases owing to welfare considerations. An exact diagnosis and a detailed explanation to the owner are essential in order for him or her to understand the prognosis and effects of the problem.

After a brief general examination the hair and skin are looked at more closely, especially areas of hair loss, loose or broken hair and skin discoloration, as well as signs of the presence of parasites, dandruff or dirt. The distribution, size, depth and spread of the lesions have to be established. Sometimes it is necessary to clip

Lumps and bumps

The numerous skin lesions have various English names and their Latin equivalents that are used as medical terms.

A few are listed below:

• **Papule:** small, hard and round lesion, closed and protruding.

• **Nodule:** about cherry-sized, hard, ball-shaped, closed, can usually be moved under the skin.

• **Vesicle:** small, fluid-filled soft surface blister.

• **Bulla:** larger than a pea, fluid-filled blister.

• **Pustule:** small clearly defined lesion that contains pus, similar to acne. Once emptied they can still be felt under the skin. Pustules are often painful.

• **Urticaria (wheals or hives):** usually soft, not clearly defined, fluid filled. They may be only a few centimetres wide or spread over large areas.

• **Squames (scurf and dandruff):** scurf is formed by small excess skin particles, as often seen in horses suffering from malnutrition, and it appears predominantly in the mane. Scurf attracts lice.

• **Crusts:** these develop from dried secretions, for example after skin injuries.

• **Cicatrix (scar):** scars are formed from connective tissue after injuries. They involve several skin layers and are usually unpigmented and hairless.

• **Ulcer:** ulcers are moist and open, usually stretching over several skin layers. They develop when the healing properties of the skin are impaired and during various skin diseases.

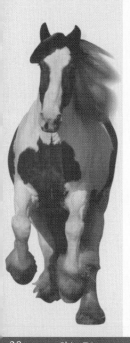

off hair or use a torch or magnifying glass. Depending on the case, walls, pastures or neighbouring horses may need to be included in the investigation.

After the visual inspection the lesions should be touched carefully to see if they are warm, moist, crusty or painful on pressure.

Sometimes the history and clinical examination are sufficient to allow one to determine or at least strongly suspect the cause. Further tests should be carried out to confirm the diagnosis. It is always important to consider the differential diagnoses – it is possible that there may be a different, similar cause. Occasionally the diagnosis can only be reached by systematically excluding all other options.

Further tests

Depending on the suspected diagnosis, hairs, crusts, skin scrapings or a biopsy may be collected for further investigation.

Except when collecting a sample to test for fungal disease, the affected area should not be disinfected before the tissue collection. For a biopsy the hair should be cut off with scissors because shaving can alter the result.

A laboratory will then check the collected material for the presence of bacteria, parasites and/or fungi. Not all viral infections can be identified satisfactorily at the moment. In addition, although some laboratories offer tests

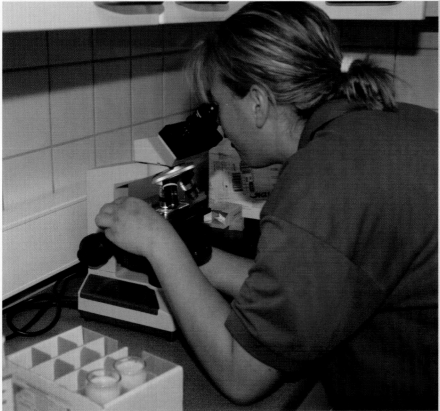

Laboratory tests can often determine the cause of the disease. (Photo: Slawik)

for Lyme disease (borreliosis) from skin samples, Lyme disease does not cause skin lesions and as such, these tests are not relevant to this book.

Biopsy

A biopsy often offers non-specific results with chronic skin diseases, long-standing injuries and secondary infections. However, in the case of acute lesions, nodules or tumours, the biopsy is one of the most important diagnostic tools. The size of the biopsy specimen (four to eight millimetres in diameter) and the location within the lesion depend on the clinical picture and suspected disease. It is often necessary to take several biopsy samples from different locations.

Use of local anaesthetic before performing the biopsy does not influence the result except when checking for mites. Performing the procedure without local anaesthetic is usually not well tolerated by a horse. It is best to use a dedicated biopsy needle because scissors cause too much tissue damage. The small incision normally heals well without needing to be sutured.

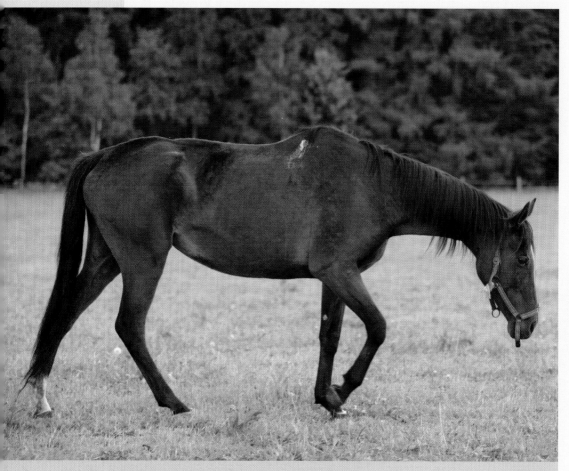

An unhealthy general appearance is often a sign of worm infestation. (Photo: Slawik)

However, when taking a biopsy from a cancerous lesion, wound healing is often considerably impaired. In these cases it is better to remove a smaller lump or tumour completely for examination.

The collected biopsy or tissue is then fixed in formalin and sent to a veterinary pathologist who will examine it microscopically to determine the type of abnormal cells and tissues. This specialised procedure is called histopathology.

Parasitological samples

Skin particles can be collected using a suction device, a hard brush or even sticky tape. Superficial skin scrapings are taken with the help of a sharp instrument from the edge of a lesion, deep enough but avoiding any bleeding. Only when testing for Demodex mites, luckily rare in horses, is a deep skin scraping needed. The collected tissue is best examined under a microscope immediately or fixated in potassium hydroxide solution. If such a sample has to be sent to a laboratory it is essential not to place it in an airtight container.

Using sticky tape for collecting skin samples from around the anus is ideal for testing for pinworm (Oxyuris equi). The worm leaves the rectum and deposits its eggs around the anus. This causes itchiness, and infected horses often rub their tails.

Bacteriological samples

Swabs or crusts sent to a laboratory can easily be tested for bacterial contamination. These samples are treated with a specific stain that makes the bacteria visible under a microscope. However, bacteria are everywhere and it is often difficult to determine whether they are the cause of a clinical problem.

When dealing with dermatophilosis (see page 28) or poorly healing wounds that require antibiotics, the bacteriological examination is of great importance. The bacteria that cause dermatophilosis sit in the crusts around the hairs and can be pulled out with the hairs quite easily. They survive for quite a long time in a sample but it is important to tell the laboratory to specifically look for dermatophilosis.

It can take up to five days for the laboratory to get the results from the samples, and even longer if a test for antibiotic resistance is required. The antibiogram tests whether various antibiotics are effective against a particular bacterium or whether the bacterium is resistant. In order to obtain a successful outcome of antibiotic treatment this test is extremely important.

Fungal samples

When a fungal disease is suspected the affected area must first be cleaned with alcohol. Some hair around the lesion is then pulled out and placed in a sterile container for transport to a laboratory.

Fungal spores in a fresh sample are not easy to find under a microscope so it is usually necessary to culture the sample in an incubator. It can, however, take up to three weeks before the fungus can be identified.

Allergy testing

For allergy testing, blood samples are taken and sent for examination. Allergies are common in horses and various 'in vitro' test kits are available in the

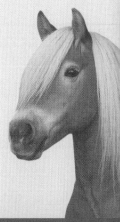

laboratory. The test agents check the reaction of specific immune cells against the allergen. Because these tests can be carried out away elsewhere the horse suffers no side effects from the tests which can also be carried out during the disease-free season.

The tests are based on immune cells found in the blood of the allergic horse. In the laboratory all other blood cells are filtered out leaving only the immune cells, the so-called basophilic granulocytes.

When an allergen that is recognised by these immune cells is added to the sample, mediators are released that can then be measured. In order to increase the specificity the test checks for only granulocytes, and only histamine as the mediator.

The test determines whether the horse is sensitised to a particular allergen and how strong the reaction to that allergen is. The more sensitised the horse is the higher the levels of histamine released, and vice versa. The test gives information on the severity of the allergy and allows grading (low grade, medium grade, severe).

Another in vitro test is also based on the sensitisation of immune cells and uses basophilic granulocytes from a blood sample as well. The cells are mixed with antigens from different insects and the levels of a mediator substance are measured, in this case a mediator called a leukotriene. The detection of which mediators allows better evaluation of an allergy is still controversial.

Both these tests require blood samples that are less than 24 hours old because their accuracy when using older blood is greatly reduced. It is also important that the cells remain intact – heat, frost or concussion destroy the cells and render the tests invalid.

There are other allergy tests on the market but they depend on short-acting free antibodies that are only present when an allergy is active, as opposed to the stable immune cells used in the more specific tests described above.

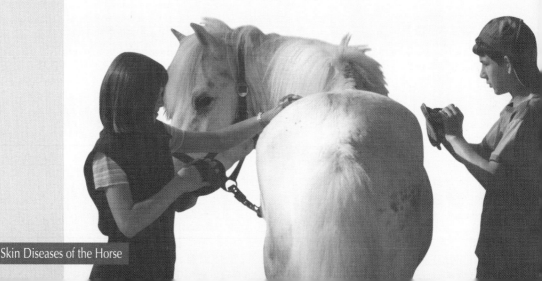

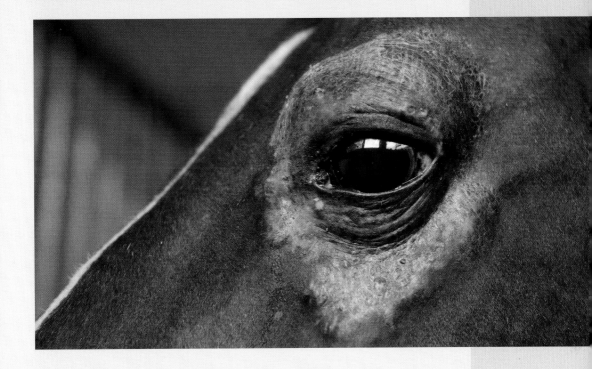

Infectious skin diseases

Viral skin diseases

Papillomatosis

This condition affects mainly young horses and foals. Suddenly the animals develop unsightly warts, predominantly around the nostrils, which can be flat and yellowish-white or more protuberant and grey. The horses are not bothered by them but of course they do not see themselves in a mirror! It is rare for these warts to be itchy.

A papilloma virus specific to horses is suspected to be the cause, although research has not been completely conclusive.

The condition usually disappears without any intervention within three months, sometimes a little longer.

Aural plaques

These bright spots inside a horse's ears are probably also caused by a virus. They develop on the inside of the ear as flat

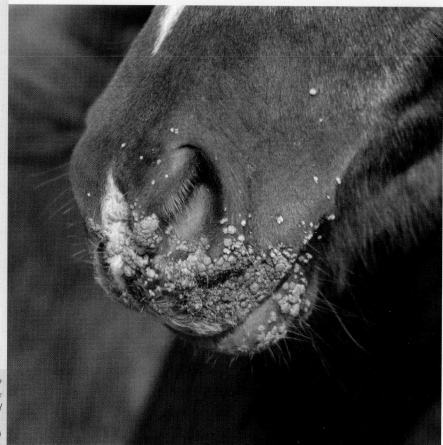

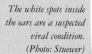

Warts that develop around the muzzle and nostrils are caused by a papilloma virus. (Photo: Stuewer)

The white spots inside the ears are a suspected viral condition. (Photo: Stuewer)

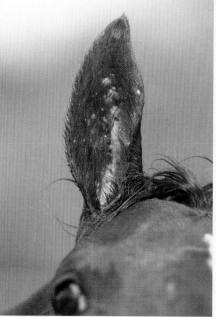

spots about one to two millimetres in diameter in horses more than one year old. They do not occur in foals. The plaques do not cause any clinical disease and will remain for life.

Pox virus

Equine pox is a rare disease caused by a pox virus specific to the horse.

The disease occurs in two variants. One form causes an uncomfortable inflammation of the mucous membranes inside the mouth, and along the borders between the mucous membranes and the skin. Small nodules appear first that turn into blisters and break open leaving wounds and crater-like lesions. Affected horses do not want to eat and produce excessive saliva. Often they also show severe conjunctivitis. The second form produces a similar inflammation in the fetlock area but it is less painful.

The causative organism is an orthopox virus. If this disease is suspected, a test for the virus should be carried out by a laboratory. The disease can be transmitted to humans and is notifiable in some European countries (but not currently in the UK).

Sarcoids

Sarcoids are benign tumours of the connective tissue that also affect the skin. They are the most common equine tumour and are most likely to be caused by bovine papilloma virus.

Sarcoids can occur in different shapes and in various body locations. Several types can affect a single horse. The tumour is invasive, which means it destroys the tissue in which it grows. Sarcoids do

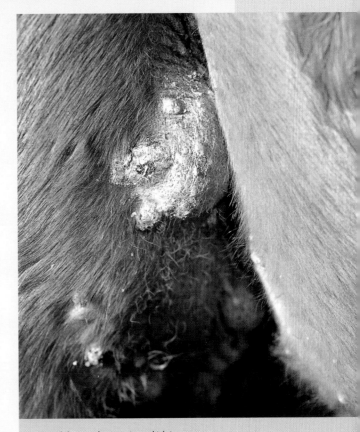

A sarcoid destroys the tissue into which it grows.

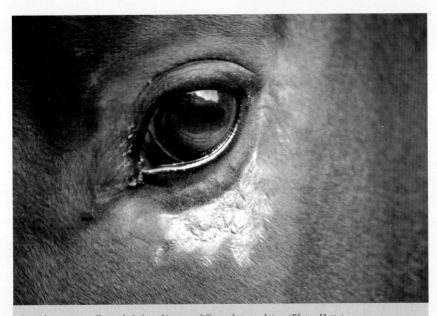

Sarcoids can appear all over the body and in many different shapes and sizes. (Photos: Hoppe)

not metastasise into internal organs and at first do not bother the horse. Unfortunately these tumours have a very high rate of recurrence: after surgical removal they are very likely to grow back in the same place. Sometimes several tumours begin to grow in different places after one has been removed from somewhere else.

There are many different treatment options. Radical removal is still the first choice and the best method – whether straightforward surgery, cryosurgery or laser therapy is used. Injection of BCG (the tuberculosis vaccine) into the tumour often achieves a reduction in tumour size, which increases the success rate of the surgery.

Every small wound sustained by a horse affected by sarcoids must be observed closely because a small wound can easily turn into a large tumour.

A susceptibility to develop sarcoids is possibly hereditary.

Vesicular stomatitis

Luckily, this disease is at present confined to the American continent. It is caused by a virus that has five different subtypes. Infected horses develop fluid-filled blisters on the mucous membranes of the mouth, on the heels and udder, and along the coronary band. The disease heals spontaneously within a short time span. Owing to strict quarantine procedures the disease has not appeared in the UK in recent years.

Bacterial skin diseases

Dermatophilosis, 'rain scald'

Rain scald is a skin disease that occurs usually during a wet late summer or early autumn. At first small hives appear underneath the skin in various places. The hair above the swelling sticks together and can be pulled out easily. The inflammation in the skin produces a fluid that dries to form small crusts. The hair in these areas can resemble a paint brush. Underneath the damaged hair the skin develops pink and moist areas but new hair will eventually grow back.

The causative pathogen is called Dermatophilus congolensis, a Gram-positive bacterium. Until the disease was identified in Europe in 1976 it was thought that this was a purely tropical condition but nowadays up to 12 per cent of skin samples show at least some involvement of this bacterium.

Dermatophilosis is often confused with a fungal infection and not treated properly. An affected horse is contagious to other horses and even humans. The bacterium cannot enter healthy dry skin, however small lesions or softened wet skin provide ideal conditions for an infection to take hold. The skin lesions do not cause pain or itchiness.

In order to confirm the disease a hair sample has to be sent off for examination. It is important to tell the laboratory that dermatophilosis is suspected so that they prepare the correct culture. Before treatment, all crusts should be removed as much as possible, but be careful because this can be uncomfortable for the horse, and wear gloves to avoid infection. It is best to soften the crusts by washing the

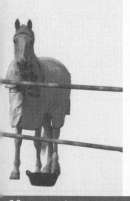

affected areas with a non-irritant shampoo. They can also be treated topically with anti-inflammatory solutions. In order to avoid further damage the skin should be kept dry with a waterproof rug. It is usually not necessary to administer antibiotics because the condition heals by itself, given good husbandry and skin care. It will disappear during the dry season anyway, but by then the horse may have lost much of its hair.

Folliculitis

Folliculitis is an infection of the hair follicles. It occurs most commonly in spring and is often located in the girth and saddle area. At first small lumps appear in the skin that can be felt with the fingers. These lumps become small pustules that open and release a watery fluid. The lesions do not itch but are tender when touched. They are caused mainly by staphylococcal bacteria, sometimes also by streptococci or corynebacteria. It is essential not to aggravate the lesions. No tack should be used and no creams should be applied. Antibiotic cream does not penetrate deeply enough to be effective; it only leads to the development of antibiotic resistance. Administering systemic antibiotics in the feed or by injection is usually not necessary. However, it is helpful to wash the lesions with an iodine-based shampoo.

The lesions usually disappear spontaneously within a few days. Once the skin is no longer tender the horse may be ridden again.

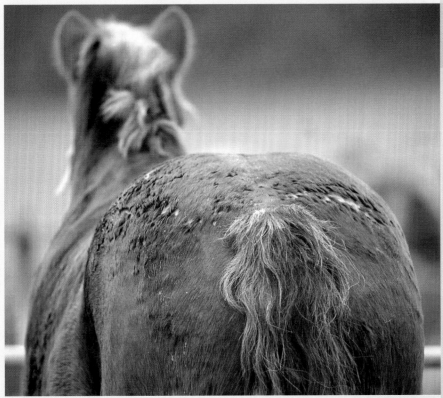

Once the skin is soaked by rain the bacteria can easily manifest themselves. (Photo: Hoppe)

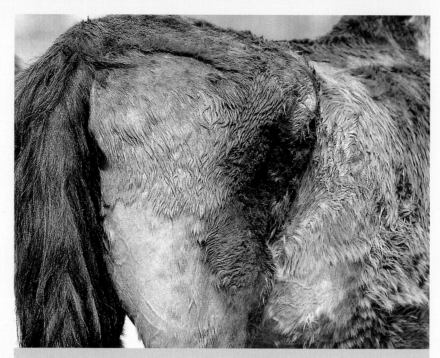

If rain scald remains untreated, large areas of hair will fall out. (Photo: Hoppe)

Furunculosis

On rare occasions folliculitis expands, destroying the follicles and involving the deeper layers of the skin. The condition becomes furunculosis, and pus-filled abscesses form. These painful lesions should be washed with an iodine-based shampoo, and a topical iodine solution should be applied. Systemic antibiotics are usually required and should be given over an extended period (at least eight days). This disease should always be treated by a vet.

Nocardiosis

Nocardiosis is a chronic skin disease manifest by hard lumps underneath the skin that appear mainly in the area of the cheeks, larynx and withers. They are neither warm nor painful. In some cases these lumps lie dormant for months before breaking open to release grey–yellow pus.

Deep crater-like wounds remain that slowly heal from the inside. The adjacent lymph nodes are always swollen.

The causative organism is called Nocardia asteroides. The bacteria penetrate the skin through tiny wounds. Cattle and dogs are much more susceptible than horses. The diagnosis is confirmed via swab or biopsy.

Some cases require surgical drainage of the abscesses. If systemic antibiotics are needed a combination of a sulphonamide and trimethoprim is more effective than penicillin. The antibiotics should be given for eight to ten days and sometimes may need to be repeated for another week. The organism can be transmitted to other horses through stable equipment and grooming brushes, therefore good hygiene is essential.

Botryomycosis

Botryomycosis is a rare chronic skin disease caused by staphylococcal bacteria that enter the skin. The subsequent inflammation shows as small pustules in the skin, inflamed hair follicles or the development of blisters. The bacteria are surrounded by immune cells and form a capsule up to two centimetres across, creating persistent swellings.

A biopsy will confirm the diagnosis. Surgical removal of the lumps seems to be the only successful treatment, followed by antiseptic and antibiotic wound treatment. Systemic antibiotics alone are often not effective because the medication cannot penetrate the capsule wall sufficiently. It is essential before using antibiotics to carry out an antibiogram because the bacteria are often resistant to various common antibiotics.

Fungal skin diseases, 'ringworm'

All fungal skin diseases that are caused by Microsporum or Trichophyton species are called dermatophytosis or dermatomycosis. These conditions often develop on damaged skin, in clipped horses or during moulting. Some of the diseases are contagious to humans as well.

Microsporosis

The first signs of Microsporum infection that are usually noticed are small hard lumps in the skin that can be itchy. After a while the hair falls out leaving circular, sometimes scurfy, areas. The affected hair breaks near the skin and can be pulled out easily from around the lesions.

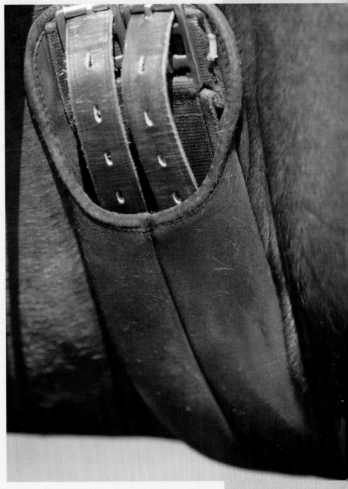

The girth and saddle areas are particularly prone to folliculitis. (Photo: Slawik)

Occasionally sticky thick crusts develop that eventually drop off leaving smooth hairless circles.

A skin scraping from the edge of a lesion is checked either microscopically or in a culture to confirm the diagnosis.

The fungal lesions should be washed with an antifungal solution (e.g. one containing enilconazole) every three days. Affected horses should be kept outside in daylight because this is the key to successful treatment. A vaccination is now available in some countries to prevent and treat fungal diseases.

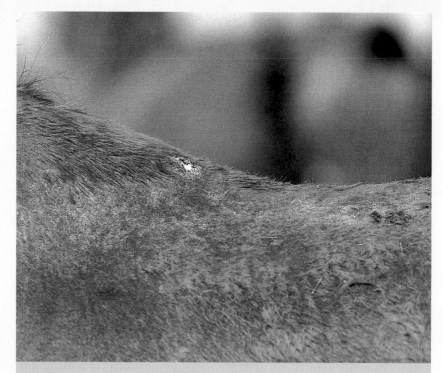

This fistula on the withers was caused by penetrating bacterial infection. (Photo: Hoppe)

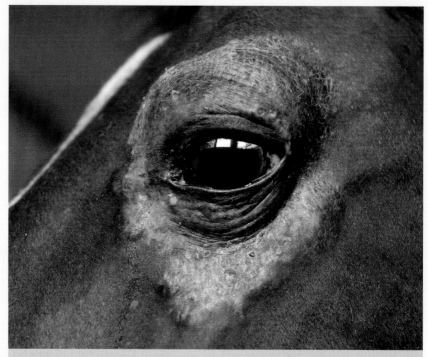

Fungal skin diseases are contagious – from horse to horse and sometime from horse to human. (Photo: Slawik)

Good hygiene is essential, and each horse should have its own grooming kit and rugs. Even spurs can transmit fungal spores, therefore the rider's equipment should be kept clean as well to avoid spreading the disease between horses. This hygiene regime also applies to vaccinated horses, because despite the protection against disease, fungal spores may still be present in the horse's coat.

Trichophytosis

Trichophyton infections are even more common than Microsporum infections and they can quickly affect a whole yard. The disease occurs predominantly in the winter and mostly affects young horses. Stress, vitamin deficiency or other underlying illnesses facilitate the infection. All body areas apart from the forehead and lower legs can be involved.

Initially small swellings can be found in the skin, rarely more than eight millimetres across, with raised hair and pale grey to yellow skin coloration.

The hair can be pulled out easily leaving bald circular areas which spread and coalesce. New hair starts to grow back in the middle of the lesions during the development of the disease, forming circular patterns. Unless the lesions become infected with bacteria they do not cause itchiness.

Microscopic examination and culture of skin scrapings will establish the cause.

The infection is best treated with diluted enilconazole solution. The first application should involve the whole body and after that the affected areas should be washed four times every three days. Washing the lesions is time consuming and prevention is always better than treatment.

After Trichophyton infection, the horse develops immunity that can last up to three years before it is susceptible to repeat infections.

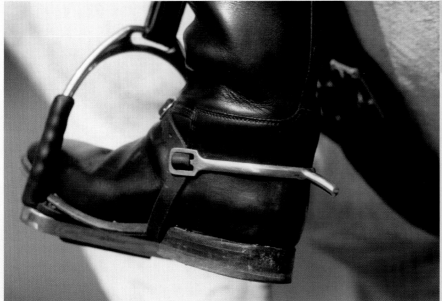

Don't forget: boots and spurs can also transmit fungal spores from one horse to another. (Photo: Stuewer)

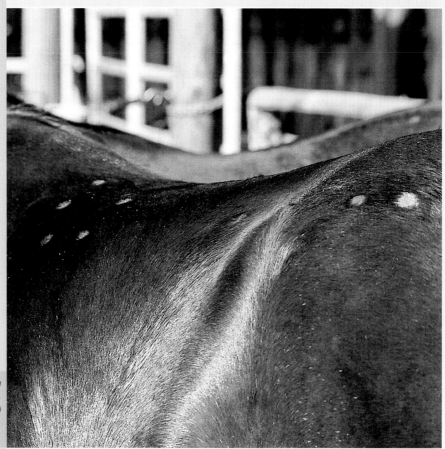

*A typical fungal infection
with circular bald areas.
(Photo: Hoppe)*

Ectoparasites

One of the most important skin diseases caused by ectoparasites is sweet itch, which is associated with exposure to midges, but this condition will be discussed in the chapter referring to immunological diseases. Other ectoparasites that cause skin problems are lice, mites and ticks.

Lice

Infestation with ectoparasites usually causes itchiness and discomfort as well as changes to the hair. A diagnosis can be reached quite easily because the parasites are often visible to the naked eye.

Lice infections are contagious and contrary to common belief, can affect even well cared for horses at times. Very young foals or older horses are prone to infestation, particularly during moulting.

Equine lice are host specific and do not affect humans. However, we can still feel itchy just from looking at them moving around the horse's coat.

Some lice infest manes and tails, feeding on dandruff. Treatment is by use of special medicated shampoos available from the vet. Lice, and sometimes even fleas, can attack any part of the body – I feel itchy now just writing about them!

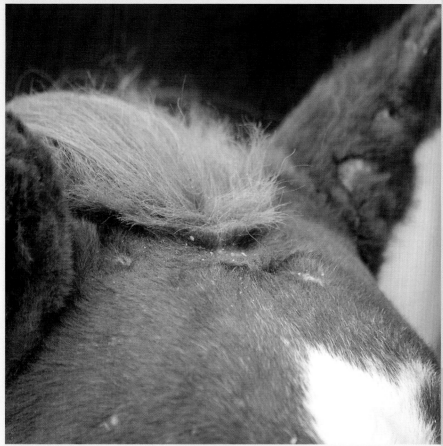

Some lice sit predominantly in the mane and feed on dandruff.
(Photo: Hoppe)

Ticks

Ticks are common visitors to the fields during the summer months. Ticks are arachnids (they have eight legs), and insecticides that act against six-legged insects are not effective against them.

Ticks live in bushes, shrubs and along the edges of forests. If you find a tick on your horse remove it immediately with special forceps or hooks, or just with your fingernails. The ticks should be removed completely and should not be treated beforehand.

Tick bites can sometimes swell up dramatically. The homoeopathic remedies Ledum and Apis can help prevent this

(get advice from a homoeopathic vet). Ticks can carry the bacterium Borrelia burgdorferi that causes Lyme disease (borreliosis), and they also carry rickettsia in certain countries, which causes ehrlichiosis. There are no satisfactory treatments for these diseases in horses, therefore minimising exposure to ticks and their immediate removal are very important.

Should your horse develop clinical signs such as apathy, loss of appetite or fever even weeks after a tick bite, you should definitely mention the bite to your vet.

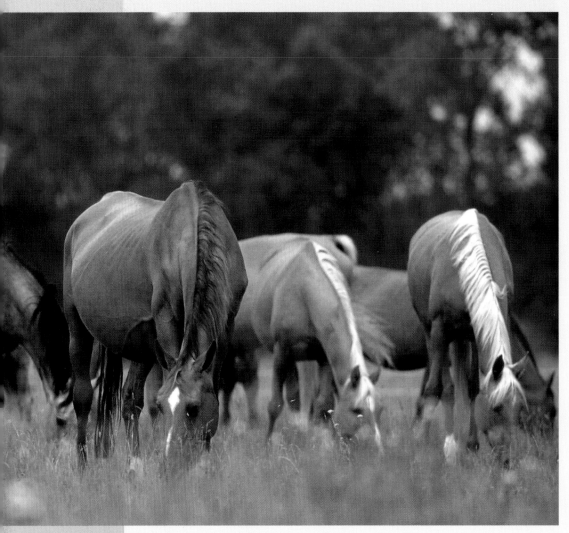

Mites

Mites living in the skin can cause mange. Three types of mites affect horses: Psoroptes, Chorioptes and Sarcoptes. All mites are arachnids (they have eight legs) and are therefore not affected by insecticides aimed at six-legged insects. All three types of mite can be detected by skin biopsy. It is important to avoid subjecting your horse to stress before a biopsy is obtained because mites are clever and will penetrate deeper skin layers when they detect stress hormones or when the blood vessels in the skin contract, which also happens in a stressful situation. The mites are much more difficult to find in such cases. The biopsy specimen must include all layers of the skin and the hair follicles.

However, the mites can often be seen when examining hair from the affected area. Most veterinary surgeries equipped with a microscope are able to obtain a diagnosis. Chorioptes mites affect the lower legs predominantly, and signs occur mainly in the winter in horses with long feathers (e.g. cobs); outbreaks during moulting are also common. Bad hygiene can facilitate the infection. The disease sometimes disappears during the summer months only to return again in the winter. The clinical signs include severe itchiness on the legs and feet, which can spread to the whole body. The skin is scurfy and tends to develop increased secretion and crusts; the hair also falls out. The horse bites its lower legs or stamps and rubs its feet. The pruritus can be so bad that the horse lies down in order to better reach its hind legs. Obviously scratching and biting only makes the condition worse. Mild cases have less pruritus and mild hair loss on the hind legs along the cannon bones.

Given that these mites generally live on the outer skin surface, mild cases can be treated with specific topical lotions. However, more severe cases require systemic medication as well, which can be prescribed by your vet.

No matter how you treat it, at best it is possible to improve the horse's condition but you will not be able to cure it completely. The mites will certainly appear again at some point, but then you know what you are dealing with and can act accordingly.

The other two types of mites usually cause much more severe and widespread signs, although milder cases are possible that are often misdiagnosed as sweet itch. The clinical signs usually occur in early spring during the moult but before the first flies appear. The mites sit deep inside the skin making diagnosis and treatment very difficult.

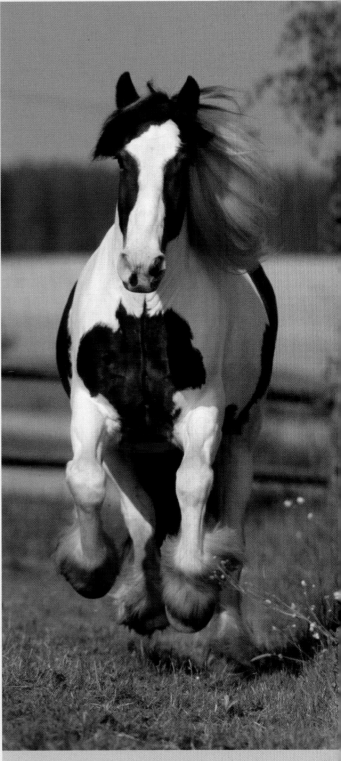

Chorioptes mites prefer horses with long feathers. (Photo: Stuewer)

Sarcoptes mites prefer areas with short hair. They cause severe pruritus, which originates on the head and spreads to the rest of the body within four to six weeks. The legs are usually not affected. Scurf and crusts appear, followed by hair loss.

Psoroptes mites affect the mane and poll areas as well as the withers and the top of the tail. Sarcoptes and Psoroptes can occur together, making obtaining a correct diagnosis even more difficult. The skin becomes scurfy and wrinkled, and prone to secondary infections.

As in cases of Chorioptes infestation, treatment is usually not completely successful but the condition can generally be improved and managed.

Endoparasites

All worms that affect horses can cause tail rubbing, especially Oxyuris equi (pinworm). This worm lives in the horse's intestines but deposits its eggs around the anus causing severe itchiness.

Summer sores

The so-called 'summer sores' are small nodules that appear predominantly on the legs and fetlocks. They are caused by a worm called Habronema, which is also a nematode. The worm finds small lesions through which it penetrates the skin, where it then deposits its eggs. Habronema larvae cause severe pruritus and

Often a sign of high worm burdens: an itchy tail.
(Photo: Hoppe)

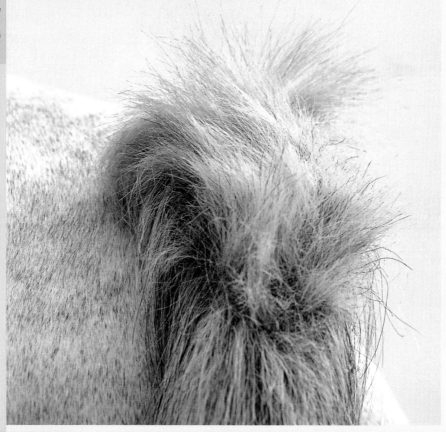

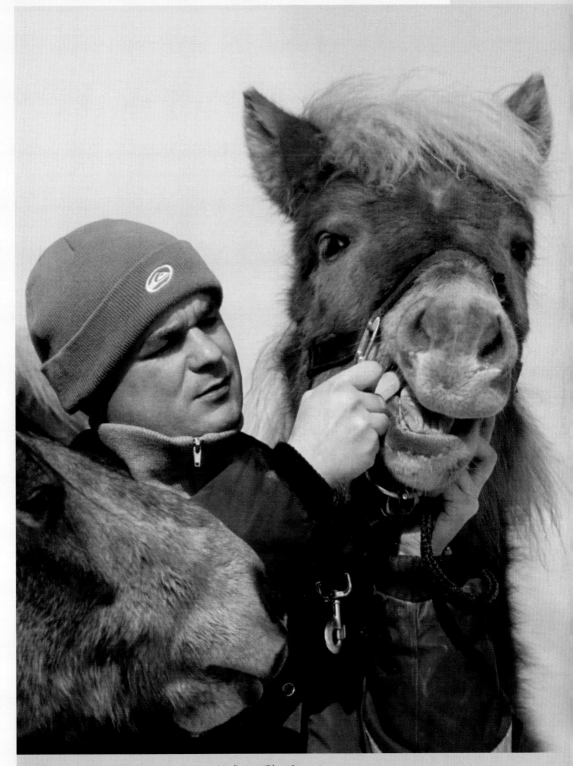

Regular worming is important to prevent serious parasitic diseases. (Photo: Stuewer)

slow-healing wounds that contain yellow–grey granules. The larvae die eventually, and the disease usually disappears in the autumn.

Onchocerciasis

The nematode Onchocerca is transmitted by biting gnats (midges) of the genus Culicoides, the same type of insect that is also responsible for sweet itch. Distinguishing between these conditions is often difficult because the insect attacks the same locations on a horse and the worms transmitted cause itchiness that resembles sweet itch.

Bots

The horse bot fly, Gasterophilus, causes eczema during the summer that is limited to the horse's head. The fly lays its eggs on the head of the horse, usually along the cheeks. The developing larvae penetrate the skin near the corners of the muzzle and spread inside the skin while sucking blood. The mechanical irritation and also metabolic products from the larvae cause an inflammatory reaction that leads to hair loss along the stripe-like pathways. The larvae meander towards the larynx where they are swallowed. The second and third phases of larval development occur in the stomach.

Eventually the larvae move towards the colon. The visible stripes on the face disappear in the autumn after the larvae have left the skin. Wormers administered in the late autumn should kill the larvae in the colon and eliminate them. If that is not the case, the larvae can lead to serious gastroenteritis, anaemia and weight loss or even death. Even a healthy horse is usually unable to cope with more than about 200 larvae (in severe cases the burden is as high as 1000 bot fly larvae in a horse).

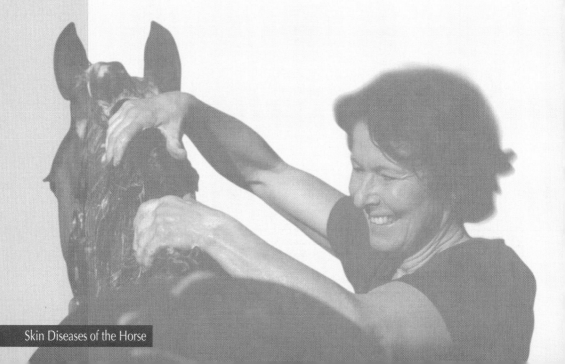

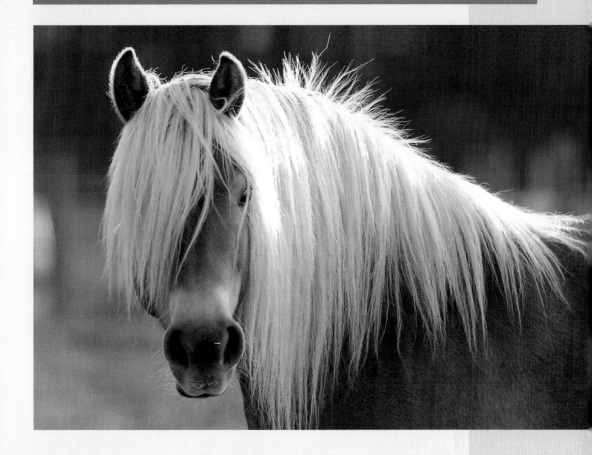

Non-infectious skin diseases

Hereditary skin diseases

A healthy skin and constitution are partly inherited, but this chapter will concentrate on skin diseases that are already present at the time of birth.

Most horses born with such problems do not live long.

Epitheliogenesis imperfecta
Foals with this condition have pieces of skin completely missing. There is no treatment. If the affected areas are only small they can heal, like wounds, to leave scars.

Congenital ichthyosis

The skin of these foals contains large areas of horn tissue, which is hairless. The foals look very scurfy. There is no treatment and these foals are usually euthanased.

Congenital alopecia

Foals with this condition are born with normal skin but without any hair. Again, there is no treatment.

Albinism

Albinism is rare amongst horses. The skin, coat and eyes lack any pigment (colour). This can affect the whole body or just parts of it.

Hyperelastosis cutis

This is a condition that affects the connective tissue. The foals are born alive, and with special care and help they can survive and have a normal lifespan. Their skin is thin and can be stretched without resistance (like a rabbit's). Such skin is more prone to injuries.

Immunological skin diseases

The two most common immunological skin diseases ('allergies') of the horse are sweet itch and urticaria. Immunological illnesses are caused by excessive or de-

A so-called 'wall eye' lacks pigment in the iris. (Photo: Slawik)

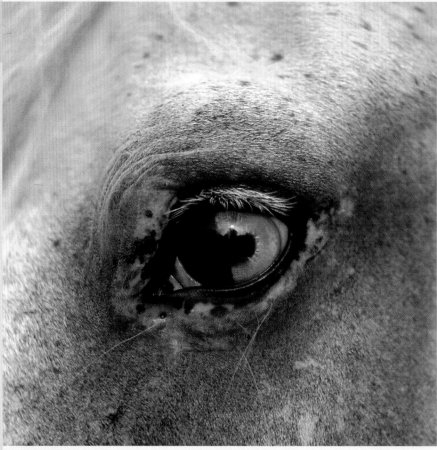

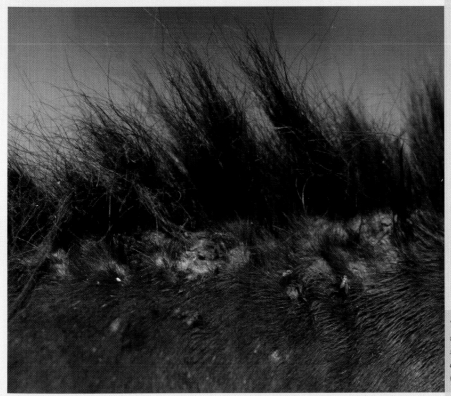

The mane has been rubbed off as a result of severe itchiness. This is a classic sign of sweet itch. (Photo: Stuewer)

fective immune reactions. The function of the immune system is to eliminate foreign agents from the body.

If the immune reaction causes a disproportionate response to an essentially harmless agent it is called an allergic reaction. Sometimes the immune system attacks substances that are not foreign but belong to the body itself. The body begins to fight against itself, thus causing an autoimmune disease.

Sweet itch

Sweet itch is an allergic skin disease that affects all breeds of horses and occurs all over the world. The allergy is caused by substances in the saliva of biting insects, mainly midges and mosquitoes. The extent of the disease depends partly on hus-

bandry procedures and the nutrition supplied to the horse.

The main clinical sign of sweet itch is pruritus (itchiness), which affects mainly the crest, abdominal midline, top of the tail, head, chest and rump. Initially, small itchy papules appear in the skin, which develop gradually into swollen crusty and sore lesions. The persistent itchiness leads to the horse rubbing these lesions. The resulting wounds are very prone to secondary infections. After years with this disease the crest is often thickened and the mane only grows back in patches.

As with all allergies, sweet itch is caused by an erratic reaction of the immune system. The body reacts excessively to contact with the saliva of the biting midges, which is the causative allergen.

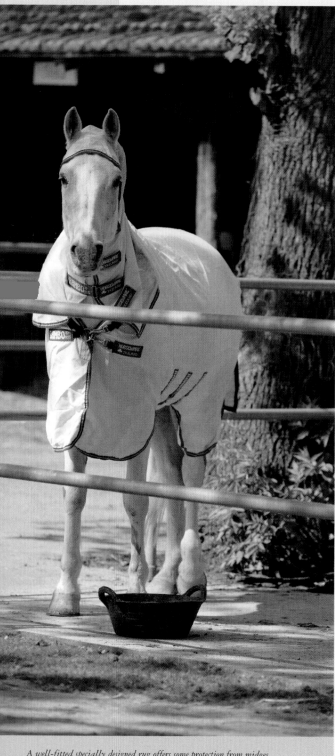

A well-fitted specially designed rug offers some protection from midges.
(Photo: Slawik)

Guard cells located in the skin of the sensitised horse recognise the allergen and release mediators that trigger an inflammatory reaction. Amongst the mediators is histamine, which is responsible for the itchiness.

A blood test can confirm a diagnosis of sweet itch (see page 23). The test measures the immune cells in the blood as well as the level of mediator substances. These specific cells remain in the bloodstream at all times, and therefore the test can also be carried out during the winter months, when the horse is free of clinical symptoms. Other tests that measure free antibodies only give a valid result during an active allergic reaction and these are also not as specific.

There is a hereditary component to this disease and it has been shown that mares are more likely to pass on the susceptibility to developing sweet itch than stallions. Despite intensive research there is still no satisfactory treatment for this condition. Every therapy has to be supported by special husbandry procedures if there is to be any hope of success.

There are three basic treatment strategies:

• **Changes to the immune system (immunomodulation).** This should be the best way to eradicate the problem at its root, but a lot more research is needed. It is possible to suppress the immune reaction, e.g. with corticosteroids, but this is short-term solution and has side effects.

• **Minimising exposure to the allergen.** Attempts can be made to keep horses and midges away from each other. This is very difficult to achieve and has several disadvantages.

• **The horse can be kept stabled all summer**, but this is not conducive to its welfare.

• **A sweet itch rug can be used**, but you must be prepared to repair it frequently and it is also useful to have a second one handy.

• **Insect repellents can be applied**, typically once or twice daily, but sometimes less often, depending on the product chosen.

• Treatment of the clinical signs. Creams and lotions that relieve the itching and encourage healing of the skin can help to alleviate the signs. It is important that the treatments are applied regularly and often.

If sweet itch is left untreated it can cause severe suffering and lead to the horse being unrideable. A complete recovery from the condition is not possible; however, special sweet itch rugs offer quite

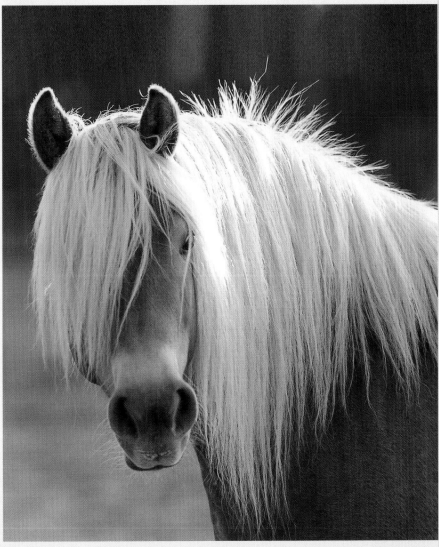

Once the sweet itch disappears in the winter the mane will grow back gradually. (Photo: Hoppe)

successful protection from midges. It is important that such a rug fits the horse and covers every part of the body, while not rubbing anywhere.

Use of the vaccination against ringworm (which is not licensed yet in the UK) has been shown to be quite successful against sweet itch. Up to 70 per cent of horses that had suffered from sweet itch for less than two years showed complete recovery, or at least significant improvement of the clinical signs, when treated as early as possible.

Urticaria

Urticaria is the most common immunological condition of the horse. It always occurs as an acute allergic reaction. Suddenly the horse is covered with lumps in the skin, usually caused by circular fluid-filled swellings (oedema), but the outer skin and coat remain intact. These oedematous areas are not usually itchy initially, but they can converge to form large wheals. If left untreated the wheals swell up more, and then break open releasing a serous fluid that forms crusts and can be itchy.

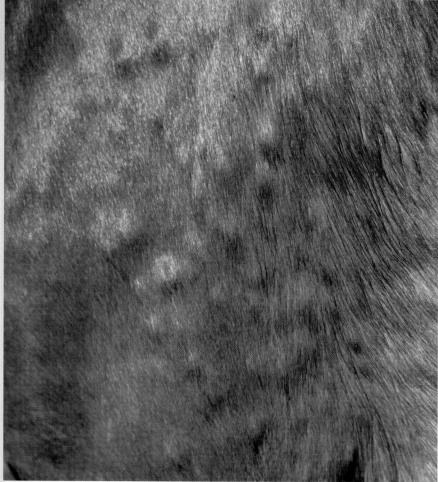

Urticaria causes lumps that spread over large areas within a short time. (Photo: Stuewer)

The allergic reaction is caused when mast cells located in the skin release inflammatory mediators on contact with an allergen. The cellular reaction is excessive, and results in the release of large amounts of mediators. The causative allergen can originate from various sources: insects, feed products, medications or infections.

It is important to try to establish the cause of the urticaria. The clinical signs usually disappear within a few hours or a couple of days. It is rare that the condition recurs or does not heal by itself, but these cases can be frustrating because sometimes not even corticosteroids completely alleviate the signs.

Normally the condition only requires treatment if the lumps break open to release a serous fluid; otherwise intervention is not necessary.

Horses can develop a very rare disease called immune thrombocytopenic purpura (sometimes called morbus maculosus). This condition also causes large wheals but, unlike horses with urticaria, which do not suffer from systemic signs, the horse will feel very ill.

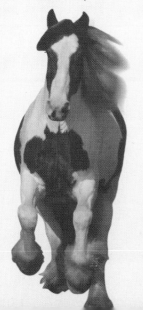

Other, possibly immunological, skin diseases

Unilateral papular dermatitis
The cause of this recurring condition is not clear. Affected horses develop small lumps and papules on one side of the body, which appear within a few weeks and usually heal spontaneously some time later.

Erythema multiforme
This disease looks similar to urticaria, with large swellings under the skin, which is thickened. The skin and hairs remain intact and do not itch. Again, the cause is unknown. This rare condition is self-limiting and usually disappears within three months.

Atopic dermatitis
Atopic dermatitis is an allergic inflammation of the skin that causes severe itchiness. It affects horses from one to six years of age. The main clinical sign is severe pruritus on the face, ears, under the abdomen and on the legs. It is usually impossible to find the causative allergen. A diagnosis is usually reached by excluding other similar diseases.

Most cases require the administration of corticosteroids in order to suppress the immunological reaction. Adding fatty acids to the feed can also help alleviate the signs.

Food allergy
Food allergies are one of the few types of allergy that occur during all seasons. Persistent itchiness that does not improve with corticosteroid medication points towards this condition. The available al-

lergy tests do not always confirm the diagnosis. To find out which feed causes the condition it is therefore sometimes necessary to remove all additional feed from the diet and then add the feed substances back in selectively. Initially only feed hay and then add different feeds to the diet. Each component should be tested for a minimum of six weeks, which makes the whole process very time-consuming. If you think you have found the causative agent it needs to be eliminated from the horse's diet for good. In order to confirm the diagnosis you can wait until the clinical signs have disappeared and then add the suspected feed to the diet again. Distinguishing between a food allergy and food intolerance is not always easy.

There is also a breed predisposition for allergies to certain feeds. Many cobs, for example, do not tolerate oats.

Some horses develop a food allergy. Excluding certain feeds systematically will finally reveal the causative substance. (Photo: Stuewer)

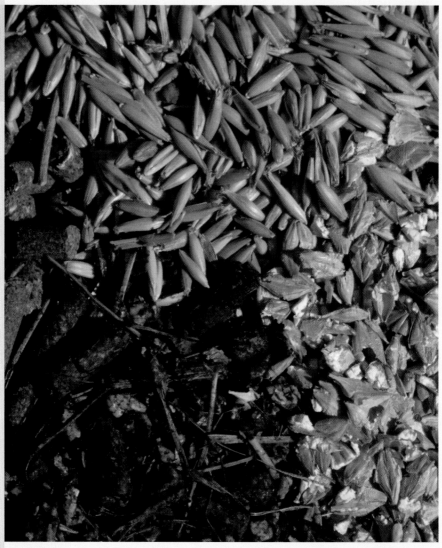

Eosinophilic granuloma

This disease is also known by the name nodular necrobiosis. It is one of the most common skin diseases seen in horses. Small lumps can appear which are neither painful nor itchy and occur predominantly in the saddle and girth areas.

The skin and hair are not damaged. The cause of these nodules, which is not yet fully understood, could be insect bites or localised trauma. Histological investigation reveals that the connective tissue is damaged and large numbers of eosinophilic granulocytes, a certain type of immune cells, are present.

A biopsy will confirm the diagnosis but often the biopsy punch leaves a wound that heals poorly. Removal of the lumps also results in a slow healing wound and the formation of scar tissue. Injection into the lesions carries the risk of infection, and the application of external solutions is ineffective.

Best practice is to ignore the lumps and leave them alone – the horse is generally not bothered by them.

Sarcoid-like dermatitis

Sarcoid-like dermatitis is fortunately a very rare disease that is usually fatal. The disease involves a typical skin inflammatory response, sometimes without systemic effects. The skin appears scurfy and crusty and the condition gradually spreads over the whole body. The hair in the affected area becomes brittle and falls out, the crusts thicken increasingly, and some horses appear lame. Treatment of the lesion will only aggravate the damaged skin. Treatment with systemic corticosteroids can help stop further spread of the disease but will not lead to recovery.

Pemphigus

This disease is caused by an immune reaction that is directed against the body's own skin cells. Affected horses usually become ill and depressed, and do not want to eat. The skin forms blisters and small lumps. The diagnosis is often problematic and depends on sending fresh blisters to the laboratory for identification. Fresh samples are sometimes difficult to acquire because the disease occurs in different phases and there are frequent secondary infections. Treatment requires long-term administration of corticosteroids at high dosages.

Immunological disease of skin vessels

This condition is relatively common and is seen only in horses. Horses of all ages can be affected, mostly during the season at pasture. Crusty, slightly swollen lesions appear along the lower legs, predominantly around white areas on the fetlocks. Removing the crusts is painful. Treatment with creams and bandages improves the lesions but will not completely cure the condition. Systemic administration of corticosteroids is recommended. Histological examination of the affected skin reveals changes to the walls of the skin blood vessels, as well as small thrombi (blood clots). It is not clear whether the condition is due to sunlight or to the ingestion of or contact with grass.

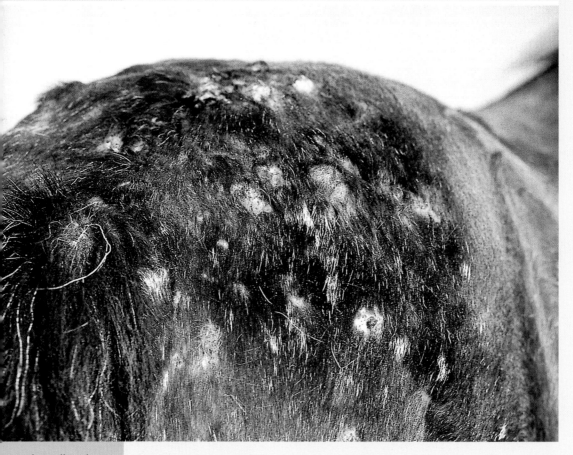

A horse suffering from pemphigus does not only look in bad condition but often also shows general signs such as inappetence. (Photo: Hoppe)

Endocrine diseases

Horses have few conditions caused by endocrine (hormonal) problems. The most important one is Cushing's syndrome – a disease caused by excess levels of the hormone ACTH from the pituitary gland in the brain. The disease has many clinical signs that are not of relevance to this book but there is also one very significant sign – hirsutism. Hirsutism is a description for the extreme hair growth and curly appearance of the coat of affected horses. Moulting is severely impaired or does not take place at all. In order to verify the diagnosis of Cushing's syndrome

the level of ACTH can be measured in a blood sample (using special tubes, techniques of sampling and a dedicated laboratory). A dexamethasone suppression test, also based on blood samples, can be used as well. Consult your vet.

Should the diagnosis of Cushing's syndrome be confirmed and the horse is otherwise well, treatment can be tried. There is no treatment for the cause; the available therapies can only limit the signs to a certain degree. The drug Pergolide is the most promising medication available currently; however, owing to the significant side effects (one of which is colic), an individual dosage must be

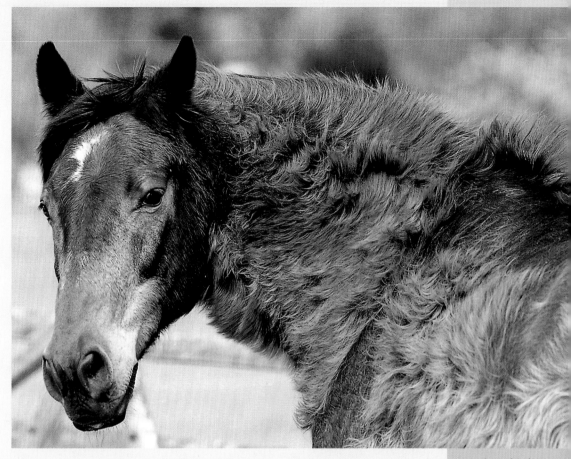

A typical sign of Cushing's syndrome is the very long coat. (Photo: Hoppe)

established accurately and frequent check-ups are required. Pergolide treatment is expensive and has to be continued for the life of the horse. Clipping the long hair will improve the horse's well-being.

Pigmentation

Albinism has already been mentioned in the section on hereditary diseases. Pigmentation problems can also occur in the form of small, isolated white spots in the coat or light transparent skin. Excess pigmentation however is very rare.

These spots are more a cosmetic issue for the owner and are not of any significance for the well-being of the horse. The medical term for white spots is leucoderma (skin without pigment), and for white hair is leucotrichia (hair without pigment).

The coats of some spotted horses appear to have a white pigment. The white areas of these horses are whiter than those of normal greys, which simply have no pigment.

Hyperpigmented spots are either congenital markings or develop after chronic inflammation or skin irritation. When identifying horses it is important

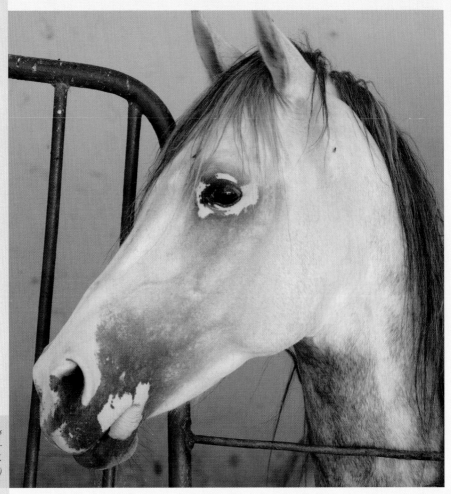

Loss of pigmentation is mainly a cosmetic problem – the horse is not affected. (Photo: Slawik)

to establish whether any markings are acquired or congenital.

Unpigmented areas develop after skin diseases, injuries, or through toxic or mechanical influences. The loss of pigment can be permanent or transient. If the hair and pigment are destroyed, white hair will subsequently grow back. Sometimes the white hairs are shorter than the normal hairs, and on rare occasions even longer. Such areas can be found as a result of saddle sores, on the lower legs after trauma, and also after freeze marking. If the deep skin layers are damaged the growth of white hairs will be life-long.

Vitiligo is a loss of skin pigment that occurs mainly around the eyes and muzzle. The cause is not fully understood. The appearance of the white areas can change throughout the season. In the case of a mineral deficiency, feed supplements may improve the condition (see the section on feeding on page 10).

Canities is the medical term for becoming grey, a sign of age in both humans and horses. Horses develop grey hair first in the area above the eyes.

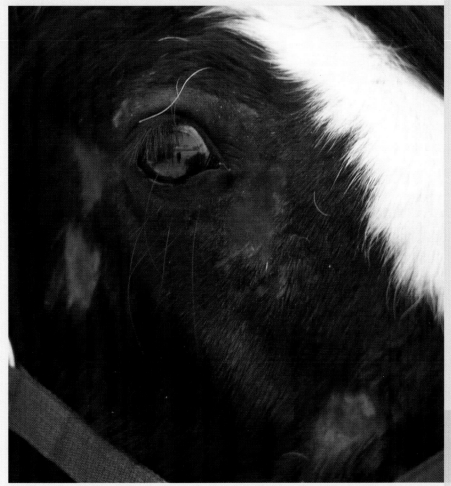

The causes of hair loss are numerous and are often impossible to diagnose. (Photo: Slawik)

Alopecia, hair loss

The simplest form of hair loss affects areas of scar tissue after injury. The hair follicles are damaged permanently and the scarred skin is unable to grow new hair.

The term alopecia also describes hair loss with intact skin, and the causes of this are unknown. Small areas can be affected (alopecia areata), but large parts of the whole body may be involved. Foals sometimes lose their baby coat before new hair has grown underneath; for a short time they are completely hairless. A condition in which the horse suddenly loses all of its hair apart from the mane and tail is called effluvium. A severe shock or trauma can suddenly interrupt normal hair development. Two or three months later new hair grows back and after the next moult the coat returns to normal. These types of alopecia cannot be treated but the horse's well-being is usually not affected. After confirmation of the diagnosis, waiting is the best and most cost-effective treatment for this condition.

Horn growth problems

Problems with keratin formation that affect the whole body are rare, but repeated trauma to an area of the skin can lead to an increase in thickness. The area of skin can become four to five times as thick and lose its hair.

Riding horses often develop typical areas of callus in the girth area, whereas trotters show them between the front legs and show jumpers around the elbow joints. These areas of increased layers of keratin are called tylomas or hyperkeratosis. They are neither painful nor warm. Once the traumatic influence is removed the skin sometimes returns to normal.

Seborrhoea

Seborrhoea is the development of crusty and scurfy skin with a greasy appearance. It is rarely a primary condition but often occurs after skin infections. The skin thickens and produces excess amounts of tallow, which then forms crusts between the hairs. The condition develops over an extended period of time. Treatment of the underlying cause and washing the affected areas with keratinolytic shampoos will encourage healing. Any kind of irritation of the affected skin must be avoided because this will increase the production of tallow again. A generalised seborrhoea that affects the whole body and has no obvious cause often does not heal.

Photodermatitis

Photodermatitis (eczema solare) is different from ordinary sunburn (dermatitis solare) because of the involvement of so-called photodynamic substances. Horses sometimes ingest such substances in the field – for example in clover, alfalfa (lucerne), vetches, beech nuts and ragwort. Horses like beech nuts and vetches, and will seek them out from the grass. Ragwort is poisonous and in grass is usually avoided. However, in hay or silage horses cannot recognise ragwort, but the poisonous properties are still active.

The photodynamic substances are transported in the blood to the skin, and sunlight will activate them in unpigmented areas, i.e. any white markings on the head and legs. This causes inflammation of the skin: primary photodermatitis.

Secondary photodermatitis can also be caused by ingestion of poisonous plants, but it starts with liver damage. The liver is unable to break down the digested plant dye chlorophyllin completely. The resultant metabolite, phylloerythrin, will increase in the blood. It is a photodynamic substance that can also cause significant skin inflammation when activated by sunlight.

When treating photodermatitis it is essential to first eliminate the cause. A blood sample should be taken in order to test liver function, and if at all possible the liver damage must be treated first. Examination of the pasture or hay is also often necessary.

The damaged skin can be treated with wound creams. Further exposure to direct

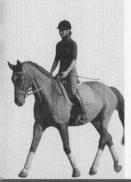

sunlight should be avoided as much as possible.

It is sometime necessary to administer painkillers. If the skin lesions are very deep, especially on the legs, antibiotics will prevent secondary infections that can easily take hold in the damaged skin.

Environmental skin diseases

Skin diseases caused by environmental influences include injuries, heat damage, frostbite and chemical contact dermatitis.

Injuries

Injuries can involve the superficial layers of the skin, e.g. a scrape or abrasion, or can cut or penetrate all skin layers. All cases lead to bleeding from the skin vessels, inflammatory reactions, release of tissue fluids, and pain.

Depending on the size and depth of the injury, surgical intervention by a vet might be required. However, natural wound healing should always be encouraged as far as possible. Suturing a wound increases the risk of infection. It is important to consider how and to what extent a wound should be treated. Sometimes leaving the wound alone is the right decision; however an initial thorough examination by the vet is always essential for a severe wound.

Applying wound cream or a bandage is often beneficial and leads to a speedier and less painful recovery.

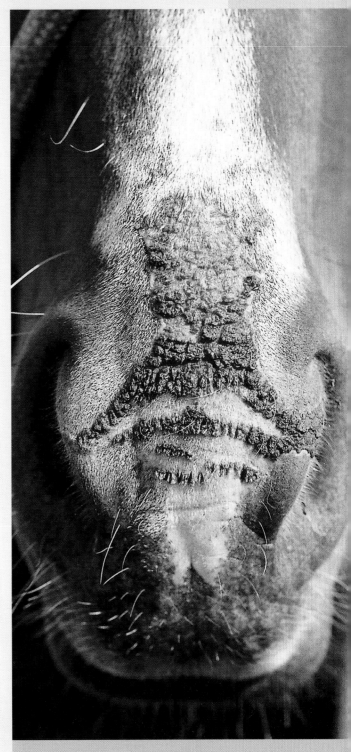

Deep sores can develop on unpigmented skin on the head or legs if horses have been sensitised with photodynamic substances. (Photo: Hoppe)

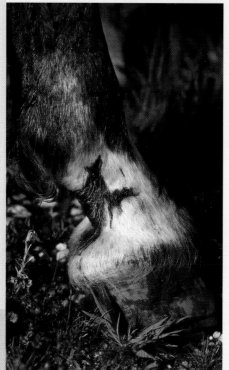

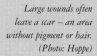

Different treatments are necessary for different types of wound. (Photo: Slawik)

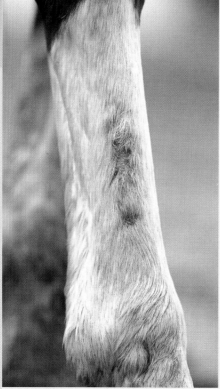

Large wounds often leave a scar – an area without pigment or hair. (Photo: Hoppe)

Different types of wounds require different interventions:

• **Abrasions** usually heal without treatment and without scar tissue.

• **Puncture wounds** have to be cleaned thoroughly and sometimes need to be enlarged in order to allow sufficient ventilation. Wounds that have airtight pockets are ideal breeding grounds for anaerobic bacteria, e.g. Clostridium tetani (the organism that causes tetanus).

• **Cuts** may slice through the skin smoothly without causing bruising or tears along the wound edges. These wounds benefit from immediate stitching, which vastly improves the healing time and cosmetic outcome.

• **Tears** rarely heal without complications, owing to the damage to the wound edges.

Depending upon the type of injury, anti-inflammatory drugs may be required. If in doubt consult your vet– better to call them too often than not enough. An up-to-date tetanus vaccination is most important for all cases of trauma.

All types of wound must be kept clean while they heal and should be observed closely for any signs of developing problems.

Common types of skin trauma, such as pressure sores from saddles or other tack, can become quite severe. An acute pressure sore looks like a closed, swollen area in the skin. The area should be cooled with cold packs or cold water. If the skin is intact the application of lotions containing DMSO®, corticosteroids or heparin can help. Any further pressure on this area must be avoided for a few days. An acute open sore has broken skin and the lesion appears warm, compressed and moist when the saddle is taken off. Within half an hour the skin begins to swell. Cooling the area is again very important, followed by disinfection of the wound and the application of creams. Pressure on this area must be avoided for several weeks, long after it has visibly healed.

The skin of a chronic pressure sore is thickened. Sometimes white hairs grow from it or it remains as a thickened area. There is no treatment for these lesions.

The damage in these cases is caused by a lack of circulation due to the pressure. The tissue dies, triggering an inflammatory reaction.

How wounds heal

Wound healing is a complex process that can be divided into three phases:

• **Inflammatory phase (demarcation):** blood and clotting substances create a crust on the surface of the wound which stops the bleeding and creates a kind of scaffolding for subsequent reactions. Immune and inflammatory cells move along the scaffolding towards the centre of the wound and remove bacteria and foreign material. Debris is also removed from the healthy tissue.

• **Repair phase (proliferation):** within 12 hours the repair mechanisms are in full swing. New connective tissue is being produced as well as new blood vessels. A thin layer of new skin spreads out from the wound edges thus initiating the third phase.

• **Final repair phase (epithelialisation and contraction):** after a week, thin pink new skin grows from the wound edges across the injured area. The wound contracts and the injured area becomes smaller. Scar tissue appears which is usually of a smaller area than the original wound. The scar tissue is not as strong and elastic as the skin and it is unpigmented and hairless. Excessive scar tissue is called a keloid. A keloid is larger than the original wound and often has a thick, uneven surface. Keloids are prone to tearing and new injuries.

Another complication common in horses is the formation of excessive granulation tissue, so-called proud flesh. Proud flesh needs to be removed either surgically or with caustic lotions.

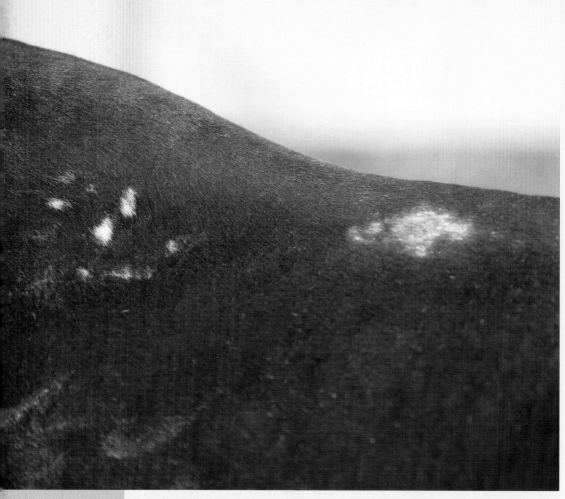

Saddle sores often remain visible for life because white hairs grow on the injured areas of skin. (Photo: Slawik)

Tack should always be well fitted and maintained. The saddle should be checked regularly to assure an optimal fit because both horse and saddle change their shape with time and may not suit each other as well as before.

The rider may also change their weight or seat at times, which may lead to variation in the distribution of pressure.

A regular check by a saddler is a sensible way to avoid saddle sores. Dirty numnahs or girths can also cause sores– as can

careless saddling and ill-fitting rugs.

Even when the best care is taken, pressure sores can occur under extreme conditions such as long distance rides, when the horse can change its shape slightly owing to the workload or through badly fitting saddle bags.

Girths that have an elasticated portion can allow a slight movement of the saddle on the horse's back, causing rub marks. Pressure sores from a tight head collar should be easy to avoid.

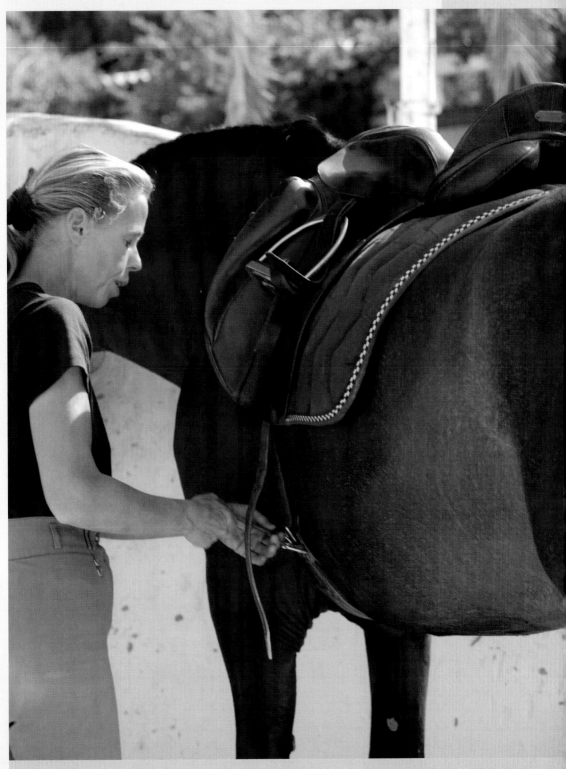

The horse should be tacked up carefully each time in order to avoid saddle sores. (Photo: Slawik)

Burns

Burns can be caused by heat, friction, chemicals or sun rays. A burn leads to temporary or permanent skin damage. Even 50 to 70 degrees centigrade will cause a leakage of tissue fluid. Temperatures of over 75 degrees centigrade will lead to tissue death.

There are four degrees of burns: first degree (combustio erythematosa), second degree (combustio bullosa), third degree (combustio escharotica), and fourth degree (carbonisation).

Burnt skin areas swell, leak fluid and lose their hair. Burns are very prone to secondary bacterial infections. It takes a few days before the extent of the damage can be established properly. Following a third degree burn, the skin dies off after about ten days leaving a crust under which new skin has already formed. It can easily take up to four months before such a burn has healed. If more than 15 per cent of the surface area of a horse has been burned, signs of shock are likely. Burns of more than a third of the body area are often fatal.

After assessment of the burn the treatment is aimed at cooling and hygiene. Ice packs wrapped in clean cotton towels are suitable. Sterile saline solution is ideal for rinsing the burnt areas. The wounds need to be covered with creams and bandages.

Friction burns may be caused by the horse slipping on concrete or damage from ropes or lunge reins. It is most important to clean these wounds carefully.

Chemical burns develop through contact with caustic substances. Such substances should never be near a horse, therefore prevention should be straightforward.

Horses that like to stand in direct sunlight instead of in the shade can develop sunburn. A shelter should be available for all horses kept outside. White areas of the horse are particularly at risk owing to the lack of pigment. Some horse owners protect the pink noses of their horses with suncream.

With all burns, the horse should be given antibiotics, painkillers and anti-inflammatory drugs. It is essential to consult a vet.

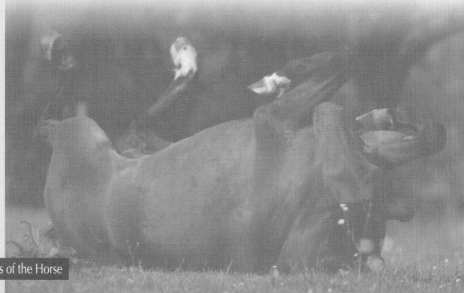

Sunburn

In the Summer, direct sunlight can cause all degrees of sunburn in areas of unpigmented skin. As prevention you need to either cover these areas or apply high factor suncreams. Once sunburn has occurred only consistent avoidance of further burning will help.

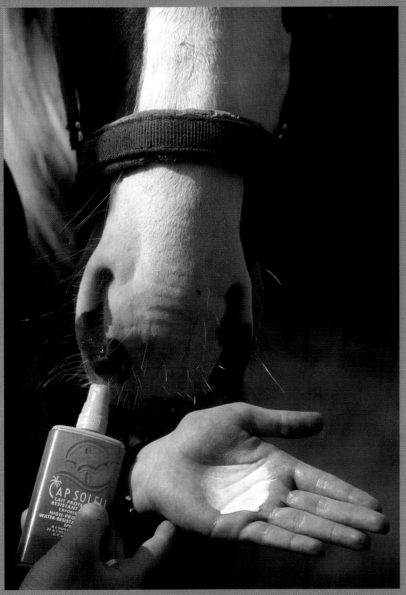

High factor suncreams can help to prevent sunburn on the sensitive white areas of the head.
(Photo: Slawik)

Pressure sores

Decubitus ulcer is the medical term for a pressure sore. Continuous pressure on a part of the body leads to a decrease in blood supply and subsequent tissue death. Horses suffering from chronic laminitis, for example, can develop pressure sores when lying on one side for extended periods of time. Bandages put on too tightly or too loosely can also cause decubitus wounds that heal only very slowly. Treatment of such wounds involves elimination of the cause, cleaning of the wound and the application of oily creams.

Contact dermatitis

Contact dermatitis is a rare event. An allergic reaction is the most likely cause. The skin changes appear shortly after new care products or fly sprays have been applied. A reaction to leather care products or a new numnah is also possible. Certain grasses or soil contaminants can cause this type of dermatitis (some horses like rolling in the left-over ashes of a bonfire, and the occasional one will develop contact dermatitis afterwards). The lesions, usually blisters or swellings, should disappear spontaneously provided the cause is eliminated.

Be careful with sprays and other products: they can cause contact dermatitis. (Photo: Slawik)

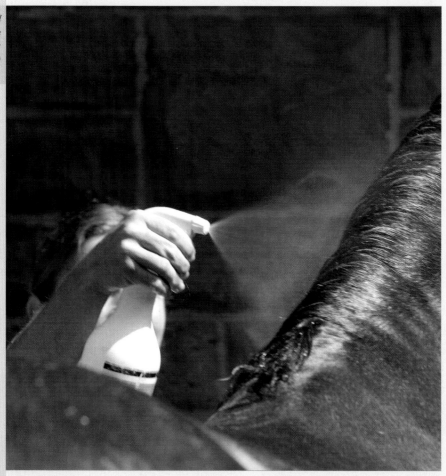

Eczema

Eczema is a term that describes skin problems such as mud fever, certain types of saddle sore, urine eczema and dandruff.

Mud fever

Mud fever is a term for various skin conditions in the fetlock area. Initially the soft skin in the fetlock area is warm, swollen and sore. The cause is a combination of a general susceptibility to external influences such as damp, dirt, or small skin lesions caused by bedding or salt grit. In the old days when working horses were fed on draff (the waste products from a brewery), the correlation between mud fever and feed was well known: heavy horses often suffered from draff mud fever.

The next stage involves invasion of the damaged skin by bacteria. This causes a persistent, multifactorial skin disease – a combination of inherited susceptibility, impaired health status, external influences and bacteria.

Horses with long feathers are particularly prone to the development of mud fever, and often mites are involved in this condition.

The mites are permanent inhabitants and cannot be eliminated completely. During moulting, when the body is under additional strain, the mites can cause disease. The lesions caused by the mites are very itchy and the horses are seen to rub or bite their lower legs and stamp their feet.

Once mud fever is established it is often difficult to treat. It often takes many weeks of intensive therapy before the skin has healed and is healthy enough

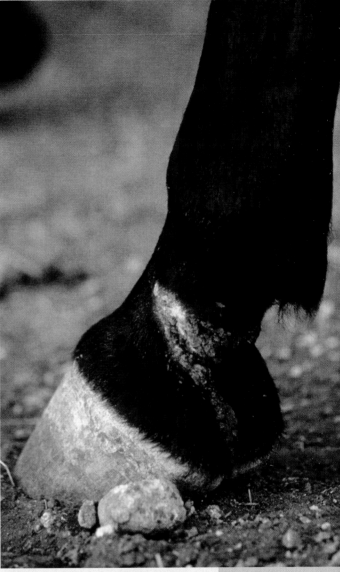

Untreated mud fever can turn into a serious disease causing lameness. (Photo: Stuewer)

to fight off bacteria. During that time it is essential that the horse is not kept in a wet stable or field.

Saddle eczema

Saddle eczema is caused by skin irritation associated with dirt and old sweat. Horses that have had a long break from work often develop this problem when first

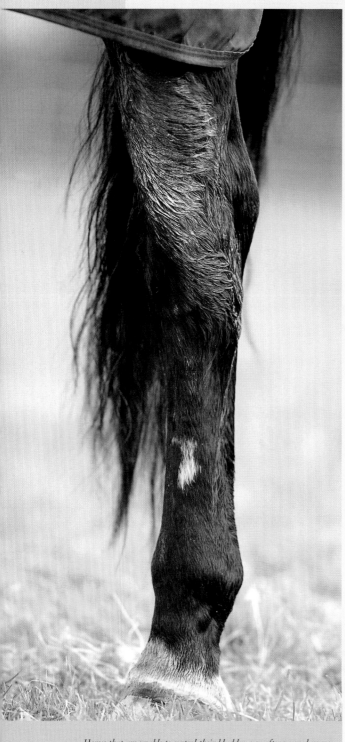

Horses that are unable to control their bladder, e.g. after nerve damage, often develop urine eczema. (Photo: Hoppe)

ridden again. Clipped saddle areas are particularly sensitive. It is not clear whether there is an allergic reaction as well. Washing the lesions with mild lotions or shampoos can help the healing process. Systemic treatment with antibiotics or painkillers is not usually required. In order to prevent this condition, using a fresh numnah every day and cleaning the saddle area carefully are recommended.

Urine eczema

Urine eczema is actually a form of contact dermatitis. Incontinence, for instance in mares after a herpes virus infection, or in horses suffering from cauda equina syndrome, can lead to permanent dribbling of urine onto the hind legs. Horses do not like this any more than people do, but in these conditions they cannot help it. The permanent skin irritation causes sores along the insides of the hind legs. The underlying problem is often impossible to rectify, therefore thorough care of the affected skin is the only solution. Depending on the extent of the lesions the use of moisturising creams or lotions may be recommended.

Matted hair

Matting of the long hair of the mane or tail can lead to a chronic skin eczema caused entirely by dirt. The hairs of the mane or tail stick together, forming dreadlocks with crusty areas underneath.

These crusts are laden with bacteria, fungal spores or parasites. A thorough wash with mild shampoo and cutting off the matted strands of hair will solve the problem.

Tumours

Tumours have already been mentioned in the section on viral diseases: sarcoids on page 27 and papillomas on page 25.

Two other types of tumour are of significance: melanomas and fibromas. Other tumours, such as lymphomas, carcinomas and lymphosarcomas, are extremely rare in horses. The causes of malignant tumours are not known. Histological examination of a surgically removed tumour or of a biopsy will usually determine the type of tumour.

Melanomas

Melanomas are mostly of a benign nature. They grow slowly and do not metastasise. It is sometimes possible for a dormant melanoma to become malignant, and thus to turn into a malignant melanosarcoma. This activation of a dormant tumour is often triggered by some kind of irritation of the tissue such as an injury. It is therefore not always recommended to take a biopsy.

Grey and coloured horses commonly develop melanomas, independent of breed and sex. The older a grey horse gets the more likely it is it to develop them. Over three-quarters of grey horses above 15 years of age have melanomas. The tumours are most commonly located in the area of the ears, around the anus, and underneath the tail.

Surgical removal of a tumour is only recommended when it becomes too large or interferes with the horse. Removal is often impossible because of the location of the tumour (e.g. too close to the veins of the ear) or the size and extent (e.g. underneath the tail).

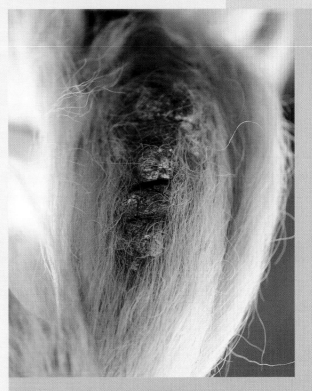

Melanomas often appear at the top of the tail or around the anus. (Photos: Hoppe)

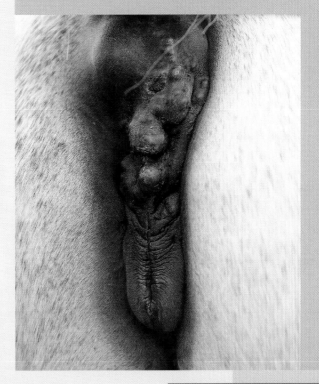

Trials with the drug Cimetidine® have only shown promise for tumours that are growing very fast. Given that melanomas usually grow slowly and do not cause pain, they are best left alone as long as they do not interfere with the horse's normal functions.

Fibromas

Fibromas are tumours of the connective tissue and can appear in any location and shape. They grow slowly, pushing the surrounding tissue away. They do not cause pain. These tumours should be removed surgically and are unlikely to return.

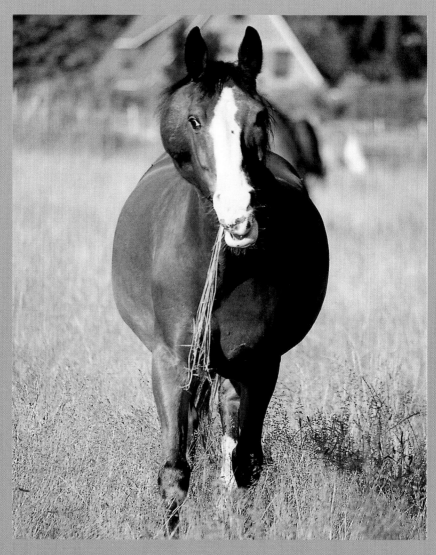

Tumours can become very large and look very sinister...

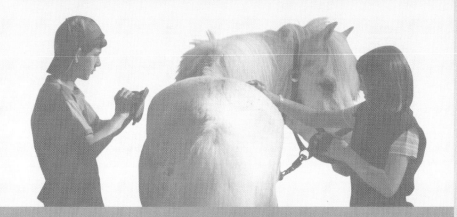

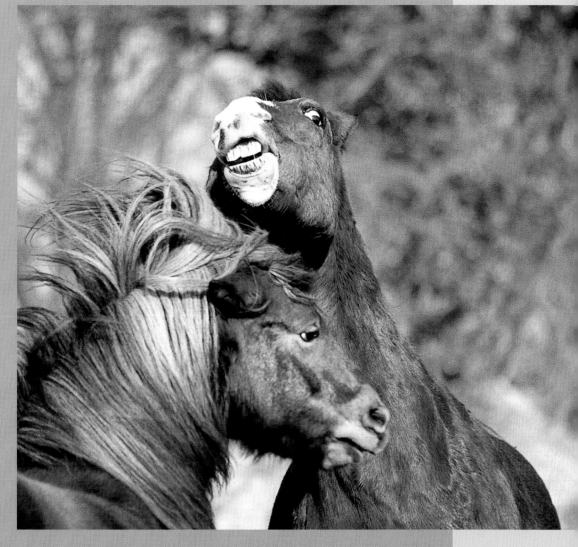

... but the quality of life, as this horse clearly shows, is often not affected. (Photos: Hoppe)

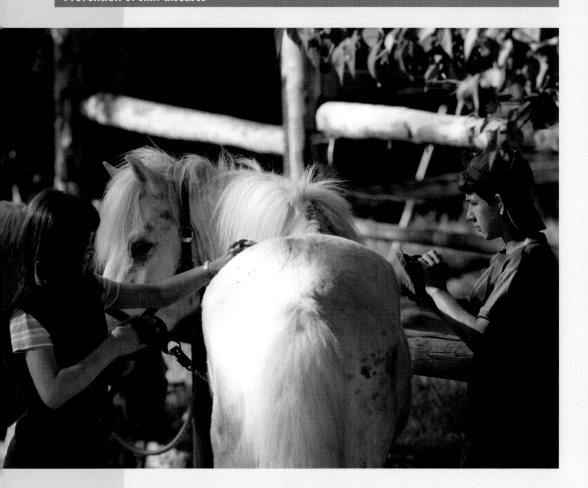

Prevention of skin diseases

Husbandry

Horses are best kept in the fresh air and with companions. At least a few hours of free exercise daily in a clean field with other horses is essential for their well-being. A 'clean field' means that all droppings should be removed at least every three days, any puddles should be drained and the left-over grass should be topped and checked regularly. Horses are flight animals and are not designed to spend much time standing around, so sufficient exercise is essential. The

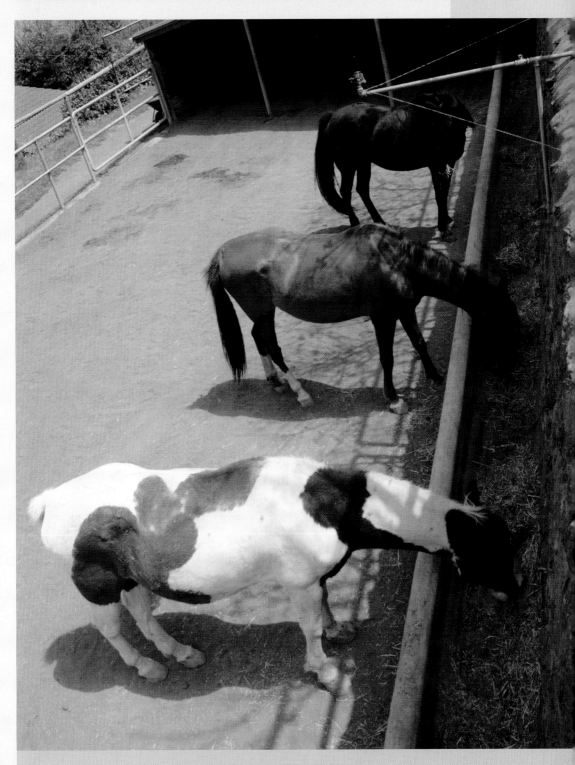

Fresh air, companions, exercise and shelter: these are appropriate criteria for good equine husbandry. (Photo: Slawik)

seasonal changes are also healthy and normal for horses. Rugging an unclipped horse is only necessary during spells of consistently wet and windy weather, and neither rain nor a mud bath does a horse any harm. Stables are best kept at the outside temperature.

Feeding

An important element of the feeding of horses – and therefore essential for a healthy skin – is sufficient roughage of the highest quality. Dusty, mouldy or otherwise contaminated hay or

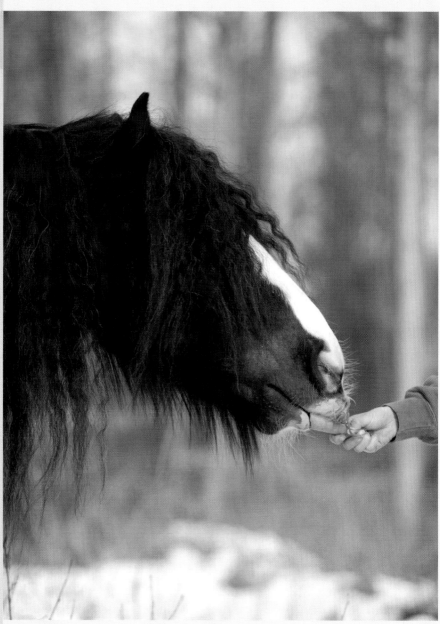

In the winter, adding feed such as carrots to the diet is recommended. (Photo: Slawik)

straw can cause serious illness. However, even the best hay cannot provide all the required vitamins, minerals, trace elements and fatty acids. A diet of just hay during the winter would also lead to a lack of energy, especially in horses that are being worked. Additional high energy feed is needed. On the other hand, overfeeding, particularly in spring, can also lead to health problems. It is then necessary to limit the grazing.

Not only what you feed the horse is important, but also how it is fed. A horse is designed to eat continuously for at least 16 hours a day while moving about slowly, but nowadays this is rarely possible. Often horses are fed three times a day with a large feed which does not take them long to ingest. Horses should spend at least six hours a day eating; breaks of more than six hours without any access to food are dangerous. At night they should always have hay or straw available to feed on.

It is best to offer roughage first and then wait a quarter of an hour before you feed the concentrate. Fresh food such as apples (a maximum of 500 grams per day), carrots or beetroot (a maximum of 1 kilogram each) are an ideal addition to the diet. You can also soak dried carrot or beetroot chips and feed them to your horse.

The teeth should be checked regularly by a trained dentist or vet and treated if required. Hooks or irregularities of the teeth lead to the horse not chewing correctly, which prevents the food being digested properly. Sharp edges along the teeth can cause injury to the membranes and significant pain.

Special feeds for healthy skin:

• **Vitamins and minerals:** biotin is known as the 'skin' vitamin. It is added to many commercial feeds and has a beneficial effect on horn and skin growth. Zinc and copper are said to be important minerals for the skin – although this has not been proven.

During moulting, any mineral or vitamin deficiency becomes even more apparent: the coat looks dull, the mane develops dandruff, and the horse is itchy and sweats more than normal. Feed supplements that are mixed in with the normal feed will help the horse during the difficult moulting period in spring and autumn. It is important to check the mineral and vitamin content of the regular diet before adding supplements because many commercial feed preparations already contain these substances and an overdose can be as harmful as a deficiency. Vitamins A, D and E dissolve in fatty tissue and can be dangerous when overdosed.

Vitamin B is important for the skin as well as the immune system. Yeast is particularly rich in vitamin B; add half a block of fresh yeast or a sachet of dried yeast to the daily feed as a supplement.

Preparations containing the minerals from algae are recommended for skin health. Many products are now available commercially.

• **Fat and oils:** plant oils are rich in energy and free of proteins, which makes them valuable additions to the diet. They also assist the body in taking up fatty acids. Different oils contain different fatty acids. Some of the fatty acids are essential, i.e. the body cannot produce them but depends on ingestion in the feed (like

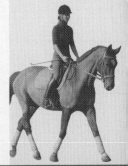

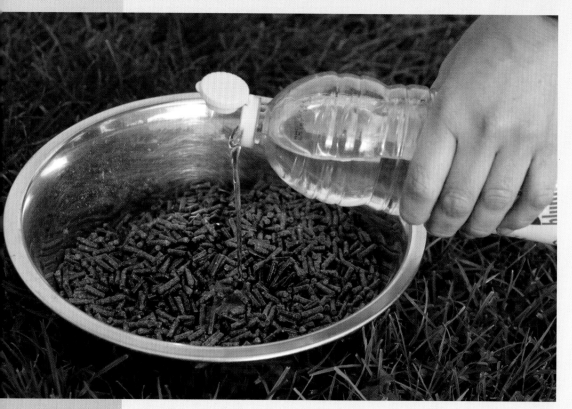

Certain oils are better than others – but adding a splash of cooking oil has a beneficial effect on the skin. (Photo: Slawik)

most vitamins that the body cannot produce itself). Essential fatty acids are important for healthy skin. Algae, fish and cod liver oil are particularly rich in these, as well as evening primrose oil, black seed oil and flax oil. Even simple sunflower oil from the supermarket can have a beneficial effect. A 'splash' added to the daily feed is sufficient. Feeding more, up to half a litre, is only useful for horses that work hard and need a lot of energy. This would be far too much for the average leisure horse.

• **Silica and sulphur:** silica is used in human products to strengthen skin, nails and hair. Silica can be added directly to the feed as a powder or you can choose a supplement that contains it mixed with other products. Many supplements

also include sulphur, which has very beneficial properties for the skin as well. It is widely used in homoeopathy for the treatment of many skin diseases.

• **Linseed:** boiled linseed is rightly called the 'wonder remedy' for healthy skin. Ideally given every other day, it also helps prevent colic, supports the metabolism and gives the horse a beautiful, shiny coat.

It is best to boil the linseed because this destroys the cyanide in it and releases the oily contents. You can simply pour 300 millilitres of boiling water over 100 grams of linseed, let it boil briefly and leave to soak for 20 minutes. The linseed does not stick to the pot then and its preparation is very easy.

Skin and coat care

Skin care for horses is a very simple affair. It is sufficient to remove dirt with a dry brush. Massages increase the skin circulation and some horses enjoy them, but you have to be careful not to remove important natural oils from the skin by grooming them too much.

Each horse should have their own grooming kit, which has to be cleaned regularly to prevent any residue from cleaning products or disinfectants remaining on the brushes. Sweat in the saddle or bridle area can be washed off with lukewarm water. A sensitive saddle area can also be cleaned with apple vinegar or alcohol. The use of shampoos is not recommended.

Small, superficial wounds can be treated with skin creams or antiseptic sprays; however, any deeper wounds that may require veterinary treatment should be left alone. Grooming sprays that make the coat shiny and help detangle mane and tail have a purely cosmetic effect pleasing to the owner's eye but they are not necessarily good for the horse. They should be used very sparingly. A horse's skin has very effective protective properties and as long as these are intact there is little for the owner to do. On the contrary: any product that blocks pores and impairs the normal functions of the skin should be avoided. Partly or completely clipped horses often need extra care in order to compensate for the loss of hair and reduced thermoregulatory ability.

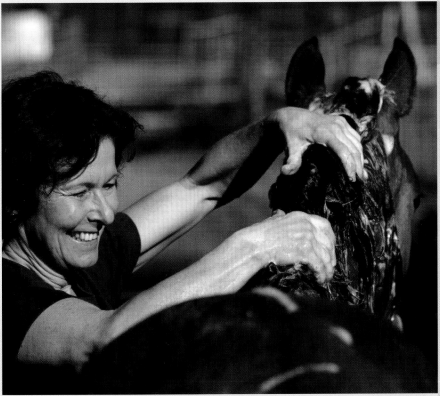

Water and shampoo should be used sparingly on horses. (Photo: Slawik)

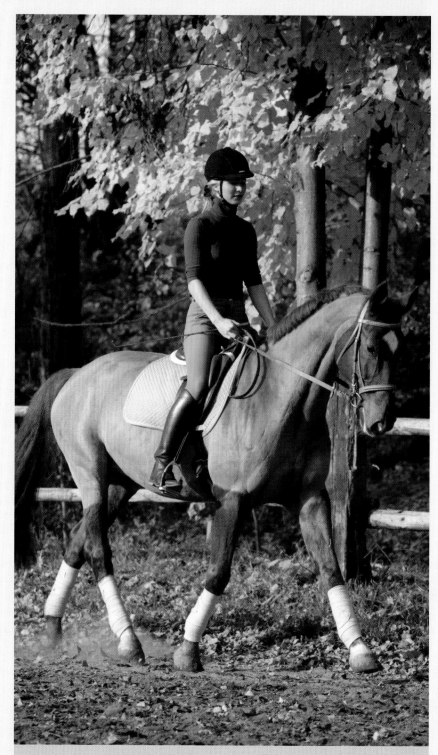

Clipping is sometimes needed to reduce sweating in horses that work throughout the winter – thermoregulation, however, will not function properly when the horse is clipped. (Photo: Slawik)

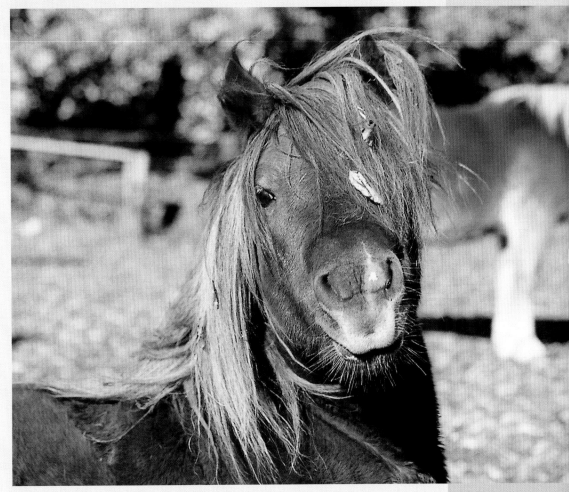

Healthy skin – happy horse. This face certainly is a happy one! (Photo: Hoppe)

Conclusion

Skin diseases in horses are a fascinating and complex subject. For some of the diseases described we have good diagnostic and therapeutic tools available. However, quite a few causes for certain conditions are still not known, and not all treatment options are satisfactory. Sometimes treatment is based on a suspected diagnosis, owing to the length of time it takes to get results from the samples collected. However, if the diagnosis then turns out to be wrong, an unnecessary, ineffective and in some cases costly therapy will have been used which could even have significant side effects.

However, although isolation of a horse, a break from its work routine and treatment of the lesions, based on a suspected ringworm infection, is annoying, it is still better than the effects of several weeks of an untreated and contagious dermatomycosis.

Skin diseases often require long-term medication and in some cases cannot be healed. It is always essential to diagnose the disease accurately so that you can ensure the best possible treatment.

Just 'putting some cream on' is not the right way forward. Often it is better to wait and learn what you can about the potential condition – which is what you have just done!

If you have a question on the subject of skin diseases you are welcome to get in touch with me via email at aruesbueldt@aol.com.

I wish you and your horse all the best.

Anke Rüsbüldt

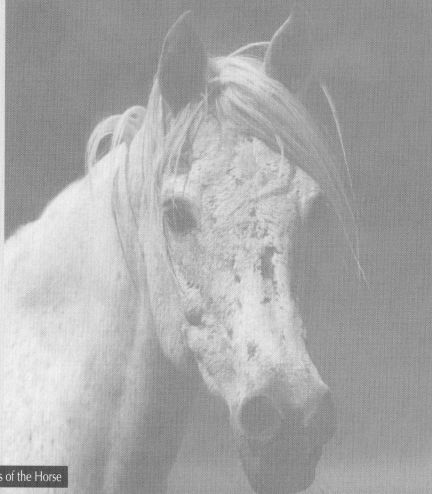

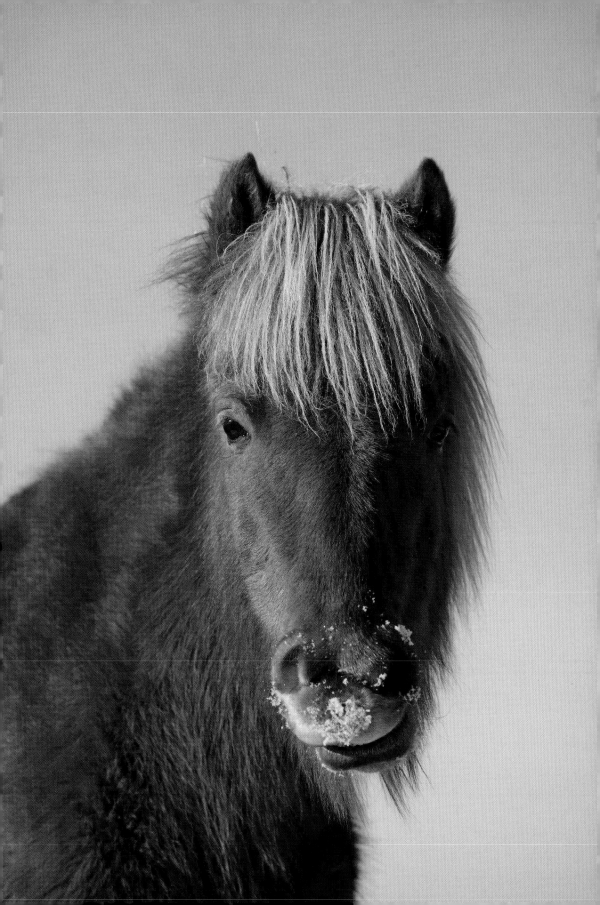

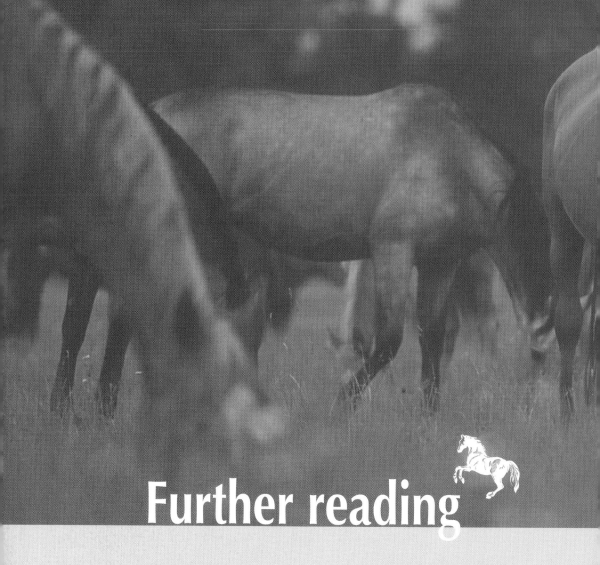

Further reading

Manual of Equine Dermatology
by Reg R. Pascoe and
Derek C. Knottenbelt
(Saunders, 1998)

**Pascoe's Principles and Practice
of Equine Dermatology**
By Derek C. Knottenbelt
(Saunders, 2009)

Practical Equine Dermatology
L. R. Thomsett
(Wiley Blackwell, 2003)

Veterinary Notes for Horse Owners
Matthew Horace Hayes
(Ebury Press, 2002)

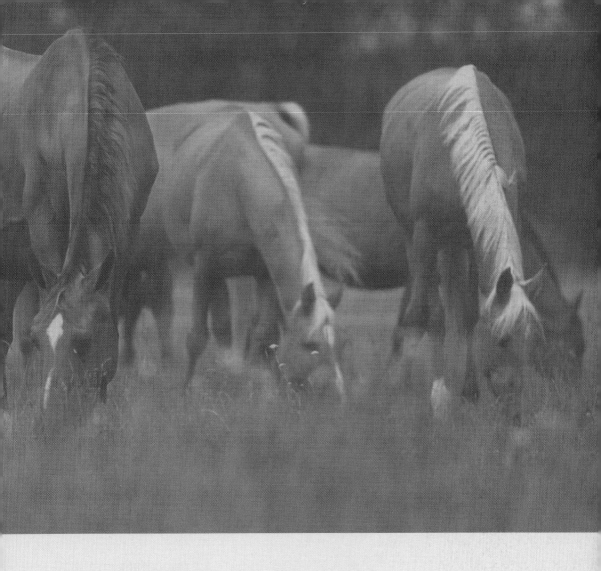

CADMOS

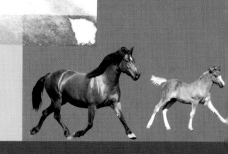

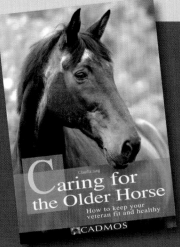

Claudia Jung
CARING FOR THE OLDER HORSE

„You are as young as you feel!" This saying applies equally to horses. Intended for the horse owner who wishes to keep his horse fit and healthy for as long as possible, this book offers an abundance of invaluable advice and recommendations – including a feeding programme, massages for the well-being of the horse, as well as age-related exercises on the ground and under the saddle.

128 pages, softcover
ISBN 978-3-86127-965-5

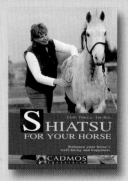

Cathy Tindall & Jaki Bell
SHIATSU FOR YOUR HORSE

In recent years, the benefit of massage, physiotherapy and other 'touch' therapies to horses has become better appreciated. Shiatsu is a traditional Japanese therapy based on pressure and stretches, the benefits of which you can share with your horse, enhancing his wellbeing and happiness. This book will familiarise the reader with the basic principals and techniques necessary to give a Shiatsu treatment that any horse will benefit from.

144 pages, hardcover
ISBN 978-3-86127-915-0

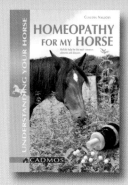

Claudia Naujoks
HOMEOPATHY FOR MY HORSE

The effectiveness of homeopathy is now taken seriously. And with a knowledge of treatments, the homeopath can help heal many common problems. However, a careful diagnosis and an understanding of the whole picture is necessary. In a very clear manner this book explains the basic knowledge necessary for diagnosis and homeopathic treatment of the most common equine illnesses.

96 pages, softcover
ISBN 978-3-86127-925-9

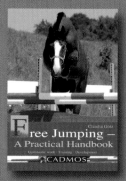

Claudia Götz
FREE JUMPING
– A PRACTICAL HANDBOOK

Most horses benefit from free jumping: It encourages freedom of movement, increases muscular strength, improves co-ordination and jumping technique. Using this practical book, which contains many helpful photos and illustrations, the reader will gain a better understanding of how to prepare for and carry out free jumping, and develop an eye for the horse's general improvement during training.

Softcover, 96 pages
ISBN 978-3-86127-954-9

CADMOS

Cadmos Books – Bringing you closer

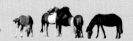

www.cadmos.co.uk